Springer Series on Child and Family Studies

Series Editor

Nirbhay N. Singh
Medical College of Georgia
Augusta University
Augusta, GA, USA

The Springer Series on Child and Family Studies addresses fundamental psychological, educational, social, and related issues within the context of child and family research. Volumes published in this series examine clinical topics with an additional focus on epidemiological, developmental, and life span issues. Leading scholars explore such factors as race and immigration, parenting, and the effects of war and violence on military families and unite a vast literature into a comprehensive series of related research volumes.

More information about this series at http://www.springer.com/series/13095

Laura Nabors

Anxiety Management in Children with Mental and Physical Health Problems

Springer

Laura Nabors
School of Human Services
University of Cincinnati
Cincinnati, OH, USA

ISSN 2570-0421 ISSN 2570-043X (electronic)
Springer Series on Child and Family Studies
ISBN 978-3-030-35605-7 ISBN 978-3-030-35606-4 (eBook)
https://doi.org/10.1007/978-3-030-35606-4

This Springer imprint is published by the registered company Springer Nature Switzerland AG
The registered company address is: Gewerbestrasse 11, 6330 Cham, Switzerland

To My Family, With Gratitude for My Parents

Preface

This book addresses anxiety and its management. The focus is on managing anxiety when a child or adolescent has a comorbid mental health problem. The first chapter reviews anxiety in children, while chapter two presents evidence-based interventions for anxiety management. Five chapters present information on mental health problems and comorbid anxiety. The mental health problems include depression, substance use, Autism Spectrum Disorder, Attention-Deficit Hyperactivity Disorder, and Conduct Disorder (defined broadly to include conduct problems, such as Oppositional Defiant Disorder). There is also a chapter on anxiety and chronic illness, as internalizing problems can be a significant issue when children are coping with chronic illnesses.

I have an interest in the treatment of children, especially elementary school-age children. However, where appropriate, literature and information for adolescents is also included. Case studies typically are presented at the end of chapters to apply information from the field. Cases are fictional and represent ideas to help clinicians working in one-on-one sessions with children. Where possible, evidence-based treatment ideas are incorporated, usually within a modular approach to addressing key presenting problems for the child. Treatment of presenting problems brings a sense of relief for the child and family and, if successful, presents a base for moving forward to intervene to address other mental health issues and family problems.

I greatly appreciate the opportunity to develop this book. The impetus for writing the book came from noticing that more information on treatment of comorbid problems in children will advance our field. The book also reflects my belief in the ability of children and families to cope with and transform their lives. Children are resilient in nature, and treatment of anxiety in the early years may prevent long-term problems. It may also reduce occurrence of other types of mental health problems.

Cincinnati, OH Laura Nabors

Contents

About the Author

Laura Nabors, Ph.D. is a professor in the School of Human Services at the University of Cincinnati. She is certified by the American Board of Professional Psychology in the area of child and adolescent clinical psychology and is a licensed psychologist practicing with children, adolescents, and their parents. She has more than 20 years of experience in research about children's mental health and providing mental health services for children and their families. This book provides insightful ideas about the treatment of children with comorbid anxiety disorders and is a tool for clinicians in a number of disciplines including psychology, social work, family therapy, and counseling.

Chapter 1
Anxiety in Children

Introduction

Anxiety is a normal response to stressful experiences and situations in the environment, and it is common in children and adolescents (Kodish, Rockhill, & Varley, 2011). From an evolutionary perspective, anxiety is an adaptive emotional reaction that leads to action that has helped our species flee, tackle danger, and survive (Vallance & Fernandez, 2016). Anxiety may be defined as, "… emotional reactions arising from … (thinking about, anticipating) … a threat to the self" (Fonseca & Perrin, 2011, p. 25). Anxiety is, "… a normal and important facet of human experience and functioning" (Vallance & Fernandez, 2016, p. 335). It is critical to normalize the experience of anxiety because mild fear is part of human development and can help humans avoid danger (Kendall, 2012). Fear is an emotional response to danger (Rosen & Schulkin, 1998). When an individual is faced with danger (or threat) there is a feeling of fear, which then dissipates when the danger decreases (or goes away). With anxiety, the emotional responses are dysfunctional and debilitating (Rosen & Schulkin, 1998).

Anxiety is a multifaceted experience for children and adolescents with somatic symptoms as well as cognitive and emotional symptoms (Kendall, 2012; Vallance & Fernandez, 2016). Children and adolescents may experience significant changes in breathing, heart rate, nausea, and perspiration rate. They may shake or cry. Intrusive, repetitive worry thoughts about what is going to happen may cognitively fuel an avoidance cycle, which further increases the child's anxiety. For example, the child may worry about a bad day at school, think about not going to school, worry more, and avoid school. The child may feel better that day, but the worry begins again that night, and can be even stronger, and in this manner the avoidance fuels and strengthens the worry. Children who are anxious in nature also may avoid things that they feel could cause their anxiety to either begin or increase in strength (Allen, Rapee,

L. Nabors, *Anxiety Management in Children with Mental and Physical Health Problems*, Springer Series on Child and Family Studies,
https://doi.org/10.1007/978-3-030-35606-4_1

& Sandberg, 2008). Exposure is important, and children need to work through their worries.

Anticipation of threat is a critical component for defining anxiety in the *Diagnostic and Statistical Manual of Mental Disorders, Fifth Edition* (American Psychiatric Association or DSM-V, 2013). Diagnosing clinical levels of anxiety occurs when the impairments interfere with daily functioning and impair relationships with others and possibly academic functioning (Garber & Weersing, 2010). Symptoms often begin around 6 years of age, although there is a wide range of ages in which symptoms occur (Merikangas et al., 2010). The most typical response to a fear-provoking situation is to avoid it (Kendall, 2012). It becomes critical to describe the reinforcement that is gained from avoiding the feared situation or stimulus to both the child and parents. A thorough explanation of avoidance behaviors helps them understand why the child needs to move through or "power through" his or her anxiety and deal or cope with feared situations and stimuli. Emotionally, the child feels fear and worry, and may sometimes describe panicking.

Prevalence

In epidemiological research, Merikangas, Nakamura, and Kessler (2009) stated a prevalence rate was 8% for anxiety disorders in children and adolescents, with a wide variation in rates of occurrence across studies. For instance, Wehry, Beesdo-Baum, Hennelly, Connolly, and Strawn (2015) report that anxiety disorders occur for about 15–20% of children and adolescents. Patel, Feucht, Brown, and Ramsay (2018) stated anxiety disorder prevalence rates vary between 10 and 30% for children and adolescents. Rates of anxiety disorders in childhood are similar to rates of anxiety in the adult years (Allan et al., 2014). Children who are sensitive to anxiety-provoking situations also may be more prone to developing anxiety disorders (Allan et al., 2014). Experts agree that anxiety disorders are the most common problem among youth (Vassey, Bosmans, & Ollendick, 2014). Generalized Anxiety Disorder (GAD) and Social Anxiety Disorder (SAD) are the most common anxiety disorders among children and adolescents (Merikangas et al., 2009). Having a comorbid mental health problem, such as depression, along with the anxiety disorder is a fairly common occurrence (e.g., Garber & Weersing, 2010). Anxiety is very serious for youth, as there is an increased risk of suicide attempts and self-harming behaviors in youth with anxiety (Jacobson, Muehlenkamp, Miller, & Turner, 2008). When anxiety symptoms are not treated, symptoms may increase over time, such that anxiety disorders persist in adolescence and adulthood (Allan et al., 2014). Anxiety disorders are related to long-term behavioral, social, and community concerns including impaired interactions with family and peers, academic problems, and substance use and other mental health problems (American Academy of Child and Adolescent Psychiatry Work Group on Quality Issues, 2007).

Anxiety disorders may be noticed during preschool or shortly thereafter. Research has shown that 9.5% of children between 2 and 5 years had anxiety disorders (Egger & Angold, 2006). For instance, Separation Anxiety Disorder, the roots of Generalized Anxiety Disorder, and anxiety in social situations are relatively common in preschool (Franz et al., 2013). Behavioral inhibition, often observed as withdrawal from interactions with peers and unfamiliar adults, exhibited by very young children can be a harbinger of later experiences of anxiety in childhood (Garcia-Coll, Kagan, & Reznick, 1984). However, encouraging positive relationships with peers and helping the child by encouraging him or her to interact with others in a variety of situations may assist with overcoming anxiety (e.g., Fattore, Mason, & Watson, 2009). Helping the child learn to regulate his or her emotional reactions, through breathing—smelling the roses and blowing out the candles—may be one method for helping the child calm down. Then, helping the child go through and face anxiety-provoking situations may teach the child a model for "powering through" situations that provoke anxiety.

There is overlap between the different types of anxiety disorders, such as GAD, SAD, agoraphobia, and Panic Disorder (Wehry et al., 2015). Anxiety is more common in girls than in boys (Merikangas et al., 2009; Patel et al., 2018). However, there are no differences in the age of onset of anxiety symptoms in girls and boys (Merikangas et al., 2009). Different types of anxiety peak at different ages with separation anxiety and phobias occurring in the younger years, while GAD typically occurs in late childhood, Panic Disorder in adolescence, and Obsessive Compulsive Disorder (OCD) in adulthood (Merikangas et al., 2009). That being said—I have treated many children with OCD and seen separation difficulties in older youth. Hence, it is beneficial to note that anxiety disorders have typical age ranges, with wide variation in ages at which symptoms are first detected and the clients present for treatment.

Characteristics

Children with anxiety disorders may be inhibited in terms of expressing emotions and may be shy and withdrawn in social situations (Essau, Conradt, Sasagawa, & Ollendick, 2012; Ollendick, Costa, & Benoit, 2010). Children with anxiety may need everything to be "just right" doing things until they are "perfect" (in their opinions). These children may therefore experience performance anxiety due to their high expectations for a perfect performance. They may also be overly concerned with how others view what they do, because they are aiming for their view of a perfect job (Essau et al., 2012). Children with anxiety may suffer from low self-esteem (Simon, Dirksen, Bögels, & Bodden, 2012). They may not have good social skills, and this and their behavioral inhibition may cause them to feel alone and have difficulty maintaining friendships (Drake & Ginsburg, 2012).

Children with anxiety often have a desire to be perfect and do perfect work, and therefore they may become upset when things are not meeting their expectation of "perfect." This desire to do everything right may result in children with anxiety being cautious and conforming to social norms (American Psychiatric Association or DSM-V, 2013). Children with anxiety disorders may be shy or socially anxious (Essau et al., 2012). This is another issue where exposure to social situations, with parent guidance and support, can help. Many children with anxiety, who are inhibited in social situations, benefit when their parents involve them in many social situations and new situations. This may assist them in becoming more at ease in the social world and in dealing with "new" or novel situations.

Several other traits are common for children who experience anxiety. Some children experience excessive, repetitive worry. The child may "ruminate" about a "worry situation" over and over, such as the child that worries about separating from his or her mother to attend school the Sunday night before the school week begins. The anxious child may tend to focus on the future and worry about what will happen in the future (Vallance & Fernandez, 2016). Teaching the child to focus on the moment and going through the next step to conquer his or her fears is important to clinical treatment. The child with high anxiety sensitivity may be fearful of new situations and people. Working with parents to help the child learn to "hang loose" and be flexible in new situations may be another component of treatment. I have helped parents determine new activities that their child can try and new situations in which the child can practice meeting other peers. Children are encouraged to join new after-school activities and attend day camps to learn to overcome fears of new situations and meeting others. Educating parents about anxiety disorders in children and adolescents is valuable, as they are treatment partners in the therapeutic process. Moreno, Furtner, and Rivara (2010) wrote a brief description as a public service for the *Archives of Pediatrics and Adolescent Medicine*, with links to the website at http://www.arhpediatrics.com, which has very helpful summary of information adapted from an article by Ramsawh, Chavira, and Stein (2010). The aforementioned article has summary information and is an example of an educational tool.

As mentioned, some children who experience anxiety, especially those with phobias, may avoid feared stimuli and situations (Allen et al., 2008). It is important for the therapist to understand root causes of anxiety. Children may need to go through the trauma of their first anxiety-provoking experiences and understand how these early experiences influence their current avoidant behaviors. Others may have high-stress lives, which has increased their tendency to be anxious (Allen et al., 2008). In these cases, children may need therapy to overcome anxiety as well as therapy to help them cope with traumatic experiences. It can be valuable to hear children's stories and allow them to voice to their feelings, as well as teach children cognitive-behavioral strategies to overcome anxiety. Children may be more likely to use the strategies if they feel "heard" and that their situation is understood by the person who is teaching them coping strategies.

Types of Anxiety Disorders

There are many anxiety disorders described in the DSM-V, such as Separation Anxiety Disorder, GAD, and social phobia (see the DSM-V, 2013). The following is a review of some common anxiety disorders:

Separation Anxiety Disorder Separation anxiety is described as being, "fearful or anxious about separation from attachment figures to a degree that is developmentally inappropriate" (DSM-V, 2013, p. 189). Children with separation anxiety can experience anxiety over separation from or loss of an attachment figure. Their anxiety symptoms may be significant in that they experience tremor, upset stomach, labored breathing, or other symptoms typically indicative of autonomic system arousal. Separation anxiety typically is present for at least 4 weeks before confirming this diagnosis (DSM-V, 2013).

Generalized Anxiety Disorder This disorder is defined as, "… excessive anxiety and worry … about a number of events or activities" (DSM-V, 2013, p. 222). The anxiety about an event, situation or thing is significant and higher than normal fear levels. The worry is often about whether or not an event or situation will occur. Children with this disorder may want to be perfect in terms of performance. Therefore, they may worry about their performance at school or for sports/activities. Children with GAD may not feel competent, experience low self-esteem, and need a lot of reassurance from others (DSM-V, 2013).

Social Anxiety Disorder Children with this anxiety problem may exhibit fear and significant anxiety about engaging in or going to social situations or social events. They may try to avoid social situations. Like children with other types of anxiety disorders, such as GAD, children with social anxiety disorder may worry about their performance and competence. Social anxiety may also include fears about being judged, watched, or excessive worry about being embarrassed (Vallance & Fernandez, 2016). They worry about how others will evaluate their performance. They may have poor social skills and few friends, and avoid seeking out friends.

Children with SAD, GAD, and separation anxiety disorder respond to similar treatments. Therapists can help them to address their fears, "power through their fears" (using graded or gradual exposure), and overcome their fears (Drake & Ginsburg, 2012). This therapist often uses relaxation and distraction for dealing with the anxiety and autonomic arousal during graded exposures to feared stimuli. Cognitive-behavioral strategies to reduce anxiety symptoms help children as they work to confront and work through feared situations, events, and experiences (Kendall, 2012).

Selective Mutism Selective mutism usually involves failure to speak in social situations where it is normal to expect a child to be able to talk with others (DSM-V, 2013). The child usually has appropriate communication skills and does not usually have speech problems. Children with selective mutism may not talk at school or in new social situations. They may selectively talk with parents or close family members. Children with this disorder are often shy and can experience significant anxiety in different types of social situations. Their parents may experience social inhibition and can be overly controlling of children (DSM-V).

School Phobia Children with school phobia refuse to go to school. They experience extreme anxiety over going to school (Maynard et al., 2015). They may have many absences and try to stay at home regularly. Children with school phobia may report they want to go to school. They just feel that they cannot get to school, because they cannot leave home. Kahn, Nursten, and Carroll (1981) defined school phobia as, "… an emotional problem, based on acute anxiety at the thought of leaving home" (p. 5).

Specific Phobia This is an excessive and persistent fear of a specific stimuli or event (DSM-V, 2013; Ollendick et al., 2015). The feared stimuli or event can be of animals; natural events in the environment (e.g., thunder); blood, injection or injury; a situation (e.g., giving a speech), or "other" type. Children with fears of specific stimuli generally benefit from gradual exposure to the feared stimuli. This allows them to confront and work through their fear of the object, as their fear is excessive and unrealistic (Ollendick et al., 2015). Vallance and Fernandez (2016) discussed simple phobias as being "… defined by excessive fear of specific objects or situations …" with subtypes relating to specific situations, animals, and nature, blood or injury, and environmental variables (e.g., water, heights) (p. 337).

Obsessive-Compulsive Disorder Children with this disorder experience obsessive thoughts and perform actions compulsively (DSM-V, 2013). Obsessions are repetitive, intrusive thoughts. Compulsive behaviors are repetitive. The child may feel compelled to perform a behavior after having an obsessive thought. The compulsion helps the child undo the worry thought and can be like rituals that the child performs repeatedly. Performing the compulsive behavior allows the child to relieve stress caused by obsessive worry. The compulsive behaviors can reaffirm or reward the anxiety thoughts because the rituals relieve the stress and reinforce obsessive thinking. There are many types of obsessive thoughts. One example is obsessive thinking focused on fear of contamination, which is undone, if you will, by compulsive handwashing. It is notable that though OCD usually involves anxiety, it may not be classified as an anxiety disorder.

Clinicians typically use the criteria in the DSM-V (2013) to diagnose several forms of anxiety disorders, including phobias, GAD, Panic Disorder, agoraphobia, separation anxiety, and Selective Mutism (Creswell, Waite, & Cooper, 2014). Anxiety is diagnosed when symptoms are at a severity level to interfere with accomplishing tasks of daily living, such as functioning within the family, school, and neighborhood. Parents may need to learn about anxiety problems in layman's terms. Thus, the following descriptions of different anxiety conditions are based on how I have explained anxiety problems to parents. The following are some descriptions I have provided to parents:

- Panic disorder can involve panic attacks (shortness of breath, fainting, and a host of other symptoms), with avoidance of anxiety-provoking events or stimuli.
- Agoraphobia involves a fear of open spaces and public places.
- Phobias involve fears of specific things, like lightning, spiders, and snakes.

- Social Anxiety Disorder involves fear of social situations and may involve avoidance of school, sports, and shopping for example.
- Generalized Anxiety Disorder involves anxiety sensitivity and feelings of worry and concern about many tasks, and often involves rigid thinking and a desire for perfection.
- Separation anxiety involves a fear of being separated from a loved one; in children it can be manifested in a fear of going to school or other social events when the child has to separate from parents (often the child's mother).
- Selective Mutism involves a child not speaking, often after a period of speaking to others. It also may involve a child whispering or making mouth movements, but no sound is made.

Assessment, Medication, and Comorbidities

Experts recommend screening for anxiety in children 8 years and older. There are many wonderful tools (see Byrne, Lebowitz, Ollendick, & Silverman, 2018 for a review). I will present one survey and one interview tool in this chapter. I have had success using the *Spence Children's Anxiety Scale*, which is a free assessment tool developed by Susan Spence. This scale is useful in clinical practice both to identify anxiety and monitor the child's progress. There is a child (e.g., Spence, 1998), parent (Nuata et al., 2004), preschool scale and preschool teacher scale (Spence, Rapee, McDonald, & Ingram, 2001) available at https://www.scaswebsite.com/. At the website, there are tabs with norms for each scale, and there are links to articles using the scales. For the child scale, children between the ages of 7 or 8 and 18 years respond to 38 questions. Children rate how much they worry and feel afraid being at home, taking a test, being alone, and so on, on four-point scales from "never" to "always." On the parent scale there are similar items. Parents rate their child's worries on the same type of four-point scale. There are items where a parent rates if their child worries and then rate specific worries, such as being away from parents, doing well on tests, and so on. There are also items that assess for physical symptoms, such as, "your child's heart starting to beat fast or your child is feeling faint."

For the preschool scales (Spence et al., 2001; https://www.scaswebsite.com/), parents and teachers rate items on five-point scales, ranging from "not at all true" to "very often true." Parents report whether their child worries about them, doing specific activities (like swimming), or is distressed about going to preschool or staying with a babysitter, and so on. Preschool teachers provide information about whether the child is able to speak in front of others, present at show and tell, exhibits worries, and so on. There are questions assessing compulsive behaviors on the Spence Scales, which according to the DSM-V (2013) might be classified as obsessive-compulsive disorder symptoms, which may be a separate disorder (no longer classified with anxiety, DSM-V, 2013). Despite this change in the most recent diagnostic manual, the Spence Scales remain valuable and free tools to assess anxiety in children and track their progress over the course of therapy.

Interviews are another tool for diagnosing anxiety disorders. For instance, the *Anxiety Disorders Interview Schedule* (*ADIS-C/P*) was developed by Silverman and Albano (1996) and has a parent and child version to assess anxiety, mood, and mental health problems in children and adolescents. Clinicians rate the severity of impairment on behavioral markers of anxiety and other behavioral problems, with a rating of four or higher indicating clinical symptoms at a level consistent with a diagnosis in the *Diagnostic and Statistical Manual of Mental Disorders*. One problem is that this scale was developed based on an earlier version of the *Diagnostic and Statistical Manual of Mental Disorders*. In the newer version of this diagnostic manual (DSM-V, 2013) Separation Anxiety Disorder and Selective Mutism have been reclassified as anxiety disorders. And, as mentioned earlier, in the DSM-V (2013), Obsessive Compulsive Disorder is separated from anxiety problems. However, I believe this rating scale can be very helpful as it has good psychometric properties and has been shown to be a good scale to use to assess change in the child over the course of treatment (Kendall et al., 2010).

A wealth of information is available about psychotherapy and pharmacotherapy as treatments for anxiety disorders in children (Patel et al., 2018; Wehry et al., 2015). Pharmacological treatments include use of selective norepinephrine reuptake inhibitors and serotonin reuptake inhibitors. Functional magnetic resonance imaging (fMRI) has shown that fear-based anxiety disorders often may be related to "... amygdala based dysfunction ..." and that other connected systems such as the "medial prefrontal cortex, anterior cingulate cortex, insula and cerebellum" may also be involved in fear-based anxiety problems for children (Wehry et al., 2015, p. 593). Kodish et al. (2011) proposed that in addition to the amygdala, the hippocampus and prefrontal cortex play a role in anxiety. Pharmacological treatments have been effective, such as fluoxetine (Prozac), sertraline, and fluvoxamine (Kodish et al., 2011; Vallance & Fernandez, 2016; Wehry et al., 2015). I have the most experience with child psychiatrists and pediatricians recommending fluoxetine or Prozac for anxiety. In my experience, it is beneficial to provide regular updates to the pediatrician about the course of treatment and to have the parents and child monitor the child for abrupt changes in mood while using Prozac. Mood swings and suicidality associated with SSRIs, like Prozac, have lessened parental preference for using this type of medication (Kodish et al., 2011). Other drugs have been examined and found to be effective in reducing anxiety symptoms in children (e.g., see Wehry et al., 2015). This therapist recommends that therapists inform pediatricians/child psychiatrists and work closely with them to determine if medication management is indicated.

Kendall et al. (2010) stated that "... anxiety disorders are often comorbid among themselves and with other disorders." For example, anxiety may co-occur with conduct problems (Creswell et al., 2014). If anxiety disorders are not treated they can herald depression, substance use problems, and suicidality in later years (Creswell et al., 2014; Kendall et al., 2010). Anxiety disorders may have a negative impact on children's involvement in family and leisure activities (Creswell et al., 2014). This book focuses on anxiety disorders and other mental health comorbidities. I do not focus on multiple anxiety disorders, although it is noteworthy that children can have several anxiety disorders or alternating anxiety disorders (e.g., Separation Anxiety Disorder can become GAD as the child becomes older). It is my belief that bringing attention to or highlighting ideas for treatment of anxiety disorders and comorbid conditions will assist with reducing the health and social burden of anxiety disorders. Many youth who experience anxiety do not receive treatment and this contributes to anxiety disorders in adulthood and the public health burden of this disorder (Creswell et al., 2014).

Cognitive-Behavioral Therapy

Cognitive-behavioral therapy (CBT) is effective in treating anxiety symptoms (James, James, Cowdrey, Soler, & Choke, 2015; Kendall, 2012). The evidence base for effective outcomes with CBT is large, whereas drug trials with children are less available (Kodish et al., 2011). I am a psychologist, with training in CBT; therefore, the case examples presented in this book focus primarily on these techniques. Some of the techniques I have modified include relaxation, positive imagery, positive thinking, use of a worry drawer, and distraction. In terms of relaxation, I work with children to teach them deep breathing. We work to blow up beach balls in our stomach to ensure that the child takes a deep breath. For young children, in order to learn appropriate breathing, we "Smell the daisy and then blow out the birthday candles." In order to relax our bodies, we practice a "rock–sponge" technique. This can be a whole-body approach or just using fists or feet. We practice making our body hard as a rock for a count of five, then we relax like a sponge and sink into the chair for a long time (in reality about a minute or so). If "rock–sponge" is done with hands, then we make a fist for a count of five, and then relax our fingers and wave goodbye to worries. If we practice with our feet, we make our feet like a rock, push the worries out through our toes and then make our feet "loose and like a sponge in a flip flop."

In terms of positive imagery, we think of a positive event, like a birthday or a trip to the amusement park and practice imagining it in detail. We think of every part of the birthday, guests coming, opening presents, blowing out the candles, eating cake and ice cream, and saying goodbye. It is important to teach children to imagine all the details, sights, sounds and smells, and so on so that the imagery can be engaging enough to interrupt or replace the worry thoughts. Other children may use iPads or computer games to distract them from their worry thoughts. As a clinician, I have learned to check with parents about whether the iPad or computer games can be used as a distraction tool. Music can be used to help distract and/or relax a child, and singing a favorite song in one's head may help the child push repetitive "worry thoughts" into the background. We talk a lot about "resetting" our systems so that the child can refocus and stop ruminating about worry thoughts. We use the strategies reviewed in this chapter to reset and defeat the repetitive worry thoughts that serve to distract from the child's "fun time."

Another imagery strategy that I use is the positive image of a superhero to combat worries. The superhero is whomever the child selects. This hero can fight the worries in any way the child likes. It may be beneficial to give the child an idea that he or she can control or defeat worries, because they can seem insurmountable. Similarly, children can use positive thinking to challenge worry statements or words they say to themselves. It is important to discuss "talking back" to worries and telling them to "get lost" or "go away." Some children, especially those who are shy and timid, may need some encouragement as they learn to talk back to their worries. After talking back to worries, then the child should replace them with positive "I can do it" statements. Additionally, the child can talk with him or herself about problem-solving steps for powering through a worry (going through the feared situation or event).

I have used a "worry drawer" with some children. For this technique a child is given some note cards or a pad of paper. The child can then write down his or her worries and worry constantly for about 5–8 min. The child should be writing all his or her worries down on a piece of paper or, if there is no paper, then talking about them and recording them on a cellular telephone (audio recording) constantly for the 5–8 min. After the time has ended, the worry notes, worry cards, or audio recording (often made on cellular telephones), should be placed in the worry drawer. A worry box (made out of a shoe box) can also be used. After the worries are placed and the drawer is shut, the child should stop worrying. The child may need to use distraction or talk back to worries, if the worries try to crowd back into his or her mind. The child should be warned that the worries may try to creep back into consciousness, and I often describe worries as "sneaky." The child needs to be a good detective to "catch" the worries and then use strategies to defeat the worries, which can interfere with fun time—a child's main job!

Distraction is often doing something fun or an alternative activity that takes a lot of concentration. Previously, I mentioned using the iPad and listening to music, which can be good distraction strategies for some children. Other strategies can be reading, playing with friends, playing a sport, or drawing. The therapist should work with the child and, if needed, the child's parents/caregivers, in order to learn what the child enjoys and becomes very involved in. These things can become distraction tools to fight against worries. Distraction is a strategy that can easily be paired with other strategies to decrease anxiety and is often a favorite for young children. If the child is not able to actively engage in a favorite distraction activity, then he or she can learn to imagine engaging in the activity (learning to use imagery to recall distracting activities may take some practice).

Case Discussion: Separation Issues and Explaining Anxiety Sensitivity

Angie is a 10-year-old girl with a history of having separation issues from her mother and being afraid of doing new things. Her therapist worked with her over four or five sessions to help her feel comfortable with coming home from school with aunts and uncles if her mother had to work late. Angie made an anxiety management book where she wrote her anxiety management strategies, such as breathing (breathe in the roses and blow out the candles on the birthday cake five times), being a rock for 5 s (holding her body tight as a rock for 5 s) and then being a sponge (relaxing her body like a sponge and sinking into her chair for a long time), or thinking of soft music to relax. She developed a strategy of talking back to her anxiety, telling it to "go away" and stop "bugging" her. Talking back to her anxiety helped her to realize that her anxiety did not have to be "large and in charge" of how she was feeling. She made a page in her anxiety management book that listed some of her favorite places to help her think of a favorite place, like the beach, or a favorite time and place, such as her birthday party at the amusement park, to block worry thoughts when they started to "take over her brain."

Angie practiced her strategies every night for 2 weeks by reading her book. She also had a reward chart, where she received smiley faces for practicing her strategies and for trying to use them when she felt worried. After every six smiley faces, Angie had "special time" to play games with her mother or father or received a sweet treat, such as an ice cream cone. Angie's anxiety went down quite a bit in the first 3 weeks, so much so that she was able to stay with her older sister without becoming scared or worried while waiting for her mother to run errands. She was able to go to school without a stomachache, which was a chief complaint she had when she first came for treatment. The therapist helped her record how much better she was feeling in her anxiety management book, and they discussed how much more fun and happy time she was having when her anxiety did not grow too large and get, "too big for its britches." The therapist described anxiety like a melting marshmallow that was "gooey" and stuck all over her brain, unless she coped with her worries and made them smaller and "shrunk them down to size."

Adults reported significant progress. For instance, Angie's mother reported higher levels of happy and bright affect at home. Her mother stated that the mornings were going a lot smoother. She and Angie were having fun during the morning, as Angie's worry about going to school and getting picked up after school decreased. Her teachers noted decreased worry in the morning. Teachers had been informed of her anxiety and its treatment. They noted that Angie was doing better at beginning assignments and focusing on work in the morning as her anxiety decreased.

By week 5 Angie's worries were greatly decreased. She was able to spend the night at a cousin's house, which was a large accomplishment. She was going to dance lessons and performed in a recital. She was nervous about performing but used her strategies and had fun doing a hip-hop dance routine with her dance class. Angie's mother reported that the chart was not being used as often, because Angie did not need it. She also was using the strategies to manage her anxiety on her own, most often challenging her anxious thoughts and thinking about her favorite places to replace anxious thoughts. If these strategies did not work, then Angie tended to move to breathing and the rock–sponge strategy. Angie had gone to a dance at her school with two other friends. Although she was nervous, she and her friends danced and had a great time.

The therapist described Angie as tending to become worried or anxious about new things and situations. She recommended that Angie and her mother might benefit from adopting a "power through" strategy to help Angie work through worry in the future. Angie's mother called a year later, mentioning that anxiety sensitivity continued to characterize her daughter. However, with continued successes and gaining more "fun time" from powering through anxiety-laden situations Angie gained confidence. She had continued to persevere and cope with being anxious about being in new situations with new people. In order to help with powering through, this therapist typically teaches the child several relaxation and thinking strategies to help the child reduce anxiety symptoms, and she often tells the child these strategies will help to reset the child's anxiety symptoms (which for some children may be an upset stomach, racing heart, fast breathing, or sweaty palms or face). The strategies help with the "reset" and then the child will need to power through his or her feared situation(s). I usually discuss powering-through fear-based anxiety, such as social anxiety and separation issues.

Because anxiety "runs" in families (genetic predisposition), parents may have anxiety (Drake & Ginsburg, 2012; McClure, Brennan, Hammen, & Le Brocque, 2001). I often invite parents to "sit in" and attend all sessions so that they can learn while their child devises strategies to manage his or her anxiety. This helped with the case of "Angie." Anxiety did "run" in Angie's family. Her mother described herself as a nervous child, and as an adult she was a "worrier." After the sessions had ended, she mentioned she might need to be referred to a clinician to address her own worries. Anxiety may be genetic and may be learned through observation of parent behavior. Parent behaviors may play a role in the development of a child's anxiety, especially if he or she models fearful behavior, and this may be especially true if mothers are anxious (McClure et al., 2001). Having parents learn the anxiety management techniques with their child may assist them to begin to address and treat their own anxiety, if they have anxiety.

Moving Forward in This Book

The rest of the chapters in this book focus on evidence-based treatment of anxiety and understanding of comorbid conditions. Children with anxiety may often have a comorbid condition or may return to therapy after a break, with another type of anxiety or another mental health problem. Thus, a goal of therapy is to offer support and strategies to win back fun time. Another is to create a warm and supportive relationship. A strong therapeutic alliance can foster the child's implementation of anxiety management strategies and provide him or her with a therapeutic atmosphere that is comfortable, making it easy to share issues with using strategies and problems coping with anxiety (Cummings et al., 2013). Moreover, this relationship is something that the child can recall and "fall back on," if he or she needs to return to therapy for a booster session if worries return or if the child needs to return to therapy to work on another mental health issue.

References

Allan, N. P., Capron, D. W., Lejuez, C. W., Reynolds, E. K., MacPherson, L., & Schmidt, N. B. (2014). Developmental trajectories of anxiety symptoms in early adolescence: The influence of anxiety sensitivity. *Journal of Abnormal Child Psychology, 42*(4), 589–600. https://doi.org/10.1007/s10802-013-9806-0

Allen, J. L., Rapee, R. M., & Sandberg, S. (2008). Severe life events and chronic adversities as antecedents to anxiety in children: A matched control study. *Journal of Abnormal Child Psychology, 36*, 1047–1056. https://doi.org/10.1007/s10802-008-9240-x

American Academy of Child and Adolescent Psychiatry Work Group on Quality Issues. (2007). Practice parameter for the assessment and treatment of children with anxiety disorders. *Journal of the American Academy of Child and Adolescent Psychiatry, 46*, 267–283. https://doi.org/10.1097/01.chi.0000246070.23695.06

American Psychiatric Association (DSM). (2013). *Diagnostic and statistical manual of mental disorders* (5th ed.). Washington, DC: Author.

Byrne, S. P., Lebowitz, E. R., Ollendick, T. H., & Silverman, W. K. (2018). Anxiety disorders in children and adolescents. In J. Hunsley & E. J. Mash (Eds.), *A guide to assessments that work* (2nd ed., pp. 217–241). New York, NY: Oxford University Press.

Creswell, C., Waite, P., & Cooper, P. J. (2014). Assessment and management of anxiety disorders in children and adolescents. *Archives of Disease in Childhood, 99*(7), 674–678. https://doi.org/10.1136/archdischild-2013-303768

Cummings, C. M., Caporino, N. E., Settipani, C. A., Read, K. L., Compton, S. N., March, J., … Kendall, P. C. (2013). The therapeutic relationship in cognitive-behavioral therapy and pharmacotherapy for anxious youth. *Journal of Consulting and Clinical Psychology, 81*(5), 859–864. https://doi.org/10.1037/a0033294

Drake, K. L., & Ginsburg, G. S. (2012). Family factors in the development, treatment, and prevention of childhood anxiety disorders. *Clinical Child and Family Psychology Review, 15*, 144–162. https://doi.org/10.1007/s10567-011-0109-0

Egger, H. L., & Angold, A. (2006). Common emotional and behavioral disorders in preschool children: Presentation, nosology, and epidemiology. *Journal of Child Psychology and Psychiatry, 47*, 313–337. https://doi.org/10.1111/j.1469-7610.2006.01618.x

Essau, C. A., Conradt, J., Sasagawa, S., & Ollendick, T. H. (2012). Prevention of anxiety symptoms in children: Results from a universal school-based trial. *Behavior Therapy, 43*, 450–464. https://doi.org/10.1016/j.beth.2011.08.003

Fattore, T., Mason, J., & Watson, E. (2009). When children are asked about their well-being: Towards a framework for guiding policy. *Child Indicators Research, 2*, 57–77. https://doi.org/10.1007/s12187-008-9025-3

Fonseca, A. C., & Perrin, S. (2011). The clinical phenomenology and classification of child and adolescent anxiety. In W. K. Silverman & A. P. Field (Eds.), *Anxiety disorders in children and adolescents* (2nd ed., pp. 25–55). Cambridge: Cambridge University Press.

Franz, L., Angold, A., Copeland, W., Costello, E. J., Towe-Goodman, N., & Egger, H. (2013). Preschool anxiety disorders in pediatric primary care: Prevalence and comorbidity. *Journal of the American Academy of Child & Adolescent Psychiatry, 52*, 1294–1303. https://doi.org/10.1016/j.jaac.2013.09.008

Garber, J., & Weersing, V. R. (2010). Comorbidity of anxiety and depression in youth: Implications for treatment and prevention. *Clinical Psychology, 17*(4), 293–306. https://doi.org/10.1111/j.1468-2850.2010.01221.x

Garcia-Coll, C., Kagan, J., & Reznick, J. S. (1984). Behavioral inhibition in young children. *Child Development, 55*, 1005–1019. https://doi.org/10.2307/1130152

Jacobson, C. M., Muehlenkamp, J. J., Miller, A. L., & Turner, J. B. (2008). Psychiatric impairment among adolescents engaging in different types of deliberate self-harm. *Journal of Clinical Child and Adolescent Psychology, 37*(2), 363–375. https://doi.org/10.1080/15374410801955771

James, A. C., James, G., Cowdrey, F. A., Soler, A., & Choke, A. (2015). *Cognitive behavioural therapy for anxiety disorders in children and adolescents*. Cochrane Editorial Group: Cochrane Common Mental Disorders Group. Cochrane database systematic reviews. New York: Wiley.

Kahn, J. H., Nursten, J. P., & Carroll, H. C. M. (1981). *Unwillingly to school: School phobia or school refusal: A psycho-social problem* (3rd ed.). New York: Pergamon Press.

Kendall, P. C. (2012). Anxiety disorders in youth. In P. C. Kendall (Ed.), *Child and adolescent therapy: Cognitive-behavioral procedures* (4th ed., pp. 143–189). New York: Guilford Press.

Kendall, P. C., Compton, S. N., Walkup, J. T., Birmaher, B., Albano, A. M., … Piacentini, J. (2010). Clinical characteristics of anxiety-disordered youth. *Journal of Anxiety Disorders, 24*(3), 360–365. https://doi.org/10.1016/j.janxdis.2010.01.009

Kodish, I., Rockhill, C., & Varley, C. (2011). Pharmacotherapy for anxiety disorders in children and adolescents. *Dialogues in Clinical Neuroscience, 13*(4), 439–452.

Maynard, B. R., Brendel, K. E., Bulanda, J. J., Heyne, D., Thompson, A. M., & Pigott, T. D. (2015). Chapter 12. Psychosocial interventions for school refusal with primary and secondary school students: A systematic review. In S. J. Wilson & C. L. Fong (Eds.), *Campbell systematic review*. Oslo: The Campbell Collaboration. https://doi.org/10.4073/csr.2015:12

McClure, E. B., Brennan, P. A., Hammen, C., & Le Brocque, R. M. (2001). Parental anxiety disorders, child anxiety disorders, and the perceived parent-child relationship in an Australian high-risk sample. *Journal of Abnormal Child Psychology, 29*(1), 1–10. https://doi.org/10.1023/A:1005260311313

Merikangas, K. R., He, M. J. P., Burstein, M., Swanson, M. S. A., Avenevoli, S., Cui, M. L., … Swendsen, J. (2010). Lifetime prevalence of mental disorders in US adolescents: Results from the National Comorbidity Study-Adolescent Supplement (NCS-A). *Journal of the American Academy of Child and Adolescent Psychiatry, 49*(10), 980–989. https://doi.org/10.1016/j.jaac.2010.05.017

Merikangas, K. R., Nakamura, E. F., & Kessler, R. C. (2009). Epidemiology of mental disorders in children and adolescents. *Dialogues in Clinical Neuroscience, 11*(1), 7–20.

Moreno, M. A., Furtner, F., & Rivara, F. P. (2010). Anxiety disorders in children and adolescents. *Archives of Pediatrics and Adolescent Medicine, 164*(10), 984. https://doi.org/10.1001/archpediatrics.2010.179

Nuata, M. H., Scholing, S. H., Rapee, R. M., Abbott, M., Spence, S. H., & Waters, A. (2004). A parent-report measure of children's anxiety: Psychometric properties and comparison with child report in a clinic sample. *Behaviour Research and Therapy, 42*(7), 813–839. https://doi.org/10.1016/S0005-7967(03)00200-6

Ollendick, T. H., Costa, N. M., & Benoit, K. E. (2010). Interpersonal processes and the anxiety disorders of childhood. In J. G. Bock (Ed.), *Interpersonal processes in the anxiety disorders: Implications for understanding psychopathology and treatment* (pp. 71–95). Washington, DC: American Psychological Association.

Ollendick, T. H., Halldorsdottir, T., Fraire, M. G., Austin, K. E., Ryoichi, J. P., … Whitmore, M. J. (2015). Specific phobias in youth: A randomized controlled trial comparing one-session treatment to a parent-augmented one-session treatment. *Behavior Therapy, 46*(2), 141–155. https://doi.org/10.1016/j.beth.2014.09.004

Patel, D. R., Feucht, C., Brown, K., & Ramsay, J. (2018). Pharmacological treatment of anxiety disorders in children and adolescents: A review for practitioners. *Translational Pediatrics, 7*(1), 23–35. https://doi.org/10.21037/tp.2017.08.05

Ramsawh, H. J., Chavira, D. A., & Stein, M. B. (2010). Burden of anxiety disorders in pediatric medical settings: Prevalence, phenomenology, and a research agenda. *Archives of Pediatrics and Adolescent Medicine, 164*(10), 965–972. https://doi.org/10.1001/archpediatrics.2010.170

Rosen, J. B., & Schulkin, J. (1998). From normal fear to pathological anxiety. *Psychological Review, 105*(2), 325–350.

Silverman, W. K., & Albano, A. M. (1996). *Anxiety disorders interview schedule for the DSM-IV: Child and parent versions*. Boulder, CO: Graywind Publications.

Simon, E., Dirksen, C., Bögels, S., & Bodden, D. (2012). Cost-effectiveness of child-focused and parent-focused interventions in a child anxiety prevention program. *Journal of Anxiety Disorders, 26*, 287–296. https://doi.org/10.1016/j.janxdis.2011.12.008

Spence, S. H. (1998). A measure of anxiety symptoms among children. *Behaviour Research and Therapy, 36*(5), 545–566. https://doi.org/10.1016/S0005-7967(98)00034-5

Spence, S. H., Rapee, R., McDonald, C., & Ingram, M. (2001). The structure of anxiety symptoms among preschoolers. *Behaviour Research and Therapy, 39*, 1293–1316. https://doi.org/10.1016/S0005-7967(00)00098-X

Vallance, A. K., & Fernandez, V. (2016). Anxiety disorders in children and adolescents: Aetiology, diagnosis, and treatment. *BJPsych Advances, 22*(5), 335–344. https://doi.org/10.1192/apt.bp.114.014183

Vassey, M. W., Bosmans, G., & Ollendick, T. H. (2014). The developmental psychopathology of anxiety. In M. Lewis & K. Rudolph (Eds.), *Handbook of developmental psychopathology* (pp. 543–560). Boston, MA: Springer.

Wehry, A. M., Beesdo-Baum, K., Hennelly, M. M., Connolly, S. D., & Strawn, J. R. (2015). Assessment and treatment of anxiety disorders in children and adolescents. *Current Psychiatry Reports, 17*(7), 591. (19 pages). https://doi.org/10.1007/s11920-015-0591-z

Chapter 2
Evidence-Based Treatments for Anxiety in Children

Introduction

There is a relatively large research base for the effectiveness of cognitive-behavioral therapy (CBT) or treatments for different types of anxiety disorders in children and adolescents (Higa-McMillan, Francis, Rith-Najarian, & Chorpita, 2016; Kendall, 2012). Several of these treatments will be reviewed in this chapter. Other evidence-based interventions will be reviewed in subsequent chapters. It is noteworthy that I take a wide-lens view of intervention approaches to include single case designs and clinical cases. Part of the reason for this orientation is based on the notion that anxiety and comorbid mental health problems may present differently across children and adolescents. Furthermore, symptoms could potentially manifest differently and respond to treatment differently when comorbid disorders are present in youth (e.g., Caron & Rutter, 1991). Consequently, learning about and gaining familiarity with evidence-based treatments for anxiety provides clinicians with a solid base of interventions from which to begin to shape programs of care for youth they serve.

Understanding the components of effective treatments and how to apply them is important, as 10% of children and 20% adolescents are likely to experience anxiety (Öst & Ollendick, 2017). Children with anxiety disorders are likely to experience other problems, such as mood disorders, other anxiety disorders, neurodevelopmental disabilities (e.g., autism) and problems with social and emotional development as well as school attainment (Higa-McMillan et al., 2016; Primeau et al., 2016; Whiteside, Deacon, Benito, & Stewart, 2016). I present a framework for using CBT techniques and applying evidence-based treatments to help children with anxiety who are experiencing other types of mental health problems. My focus remains cognitive-behavioral, with a goal of helping a child act him or herself into a new way of thinking or think himself or herself into a new way of acting. Additionally, I review specific treatment strategies, with a goal of emphasizing how they can be applied in practice using excerpts, with pseudonames, from case examples. Additionally, one

L. Nabors, *Anxiety Management in Children with Mental and Physical Health Problems*, Springer Series on Child and Family Studies,
https://doi.org/10.1007/978-3-030-35606-4_2

example of a treatment guide is entitled, *Anxiety Disorders in Children and Adolescents: Research, Assessment and Intervention*, edited by Silverman and Treffers (2001). This is a resource for learning more about interventions and tools that work with children.

Coping Cat

One of the widely known treatments for anxiety in children is Kendall's Coping Cat (e.g., Kendall, 2012; Kendall & Hedtke, 2006a, 2006b). This program teaches coping strategies through the FEAR acronym. The child is taught to recognize the bodily symptoms of anxiety—"F—feeling frightened?), by understanding his or her own physiological anxiety symptoms, such as increased heart rate and respiratory rate, and feeling dizzy. Next, the child is taught to understand his or her anxiety provoking cognitions through the "E" step—expecting negative things to happen? After this, the child is to employ coping attitudes and behaviors in the "A" step (attitudes and actions that help), such as using positive self-statements ("I can cope with my worry") and taking positive actions, such as relaxing or distracting oneself from anxiety provoking thoughts. Actions also often involve powering through or going through one's worry situation or event. The "R" involves consideration of the results achieved and rewarding oneself. Before the child goes through the FEAR steps in relation to his or her fears, the child learns positive self-statements, relaxation, and problem-solving related to his or her anxiety situation, event or object. Using imaginary modeling or through watching a role model, the child or adolescent can also visualize successfully coping with his or her anxiety-provoking situation or watch another model successfully dealing with the situation. After checking on results, the child may use self-praise or a small reward can be given for successful anxiety management. Therapists using the Coping Cat Program also use homework to help the child practice skills that he or she has learned. These homework exercises—"Show That I Can" or "STIC" exercises—allow the child to practice the techniques he or she learned in a treatment session. The homework allows the therapist to personalize the anxiety management strategies (strategies often focus on changes in thinking or behaviors to relax and reset the child's system). Thus, homework is personalized for the child's experiences and abilities (Kendall, 2012).

Older Youth: Child/Adolescent Anxiety Multimodal Treatment Study

The Child/Adolescent Anxiety Multimodal Treatment Study (CAMS) assessed outcomes for 488 children and adolescents (7–17 years) comparing the effect of CBT, sertraline, CBT + sertraline, and a placebo pill (Walkup et al., 2008). The CBT sessions lasted for 12 weeks. The Coping Cat Program was modified for this trial. Kendall is a proponent of fidelity to treatment ideas within flexible clinical administration of anxiety management tools (Kendall, Gosch, Furr, & Sood, 2008). This notion is invaluable to delivering child-focused treatment, which "fits" with the child's abilities and personal experiences. Treatment in the CAMS project focused on teaching children and adolescents a variety of anxiety management skills and providing behavioral exposure to anxiety-provoking situations. Kendall (2012) wrote that practicing skills to overcome anxiety in situations that provoke anxiety (exposures), "... provide(s) the child with opportunities to demonstrate his or her abilities in real-life situations and to develop a sense of self-competence" (p. 155). After the treatment had ended, children participated in 6 monthly booster sessions (termed maintenance treatment). The children assigned to a medication arm of treatment remained on sertraline during that time. Youth in the placebo pill condition were offered treatment, if they were still experiencing symptoms after the 12-week treatment or during the 6-month follow-up period. Results showed that the combined treatment (CBT + sertraline) showed the greatest symptom reduction and recovery for children and adolescents. Relatively few children responded to the placebo pill, indicating that children need treatment (Piacentini et al., 2014). Follow-up assessments were conducted at weeks 24 and 36 (treatment ended at 12 weeks). Most children were still responding positively at weeks 24 and 36, and, as expected, the combination cognitive behavioral therapy plus sertraline group was exhibiting the highest level of functioning, followed by the CBT only and sertraline only groups (Piacentini et al., 2014).

Parent Involvement

Anxiety disorders tend to run in families. Thus, treating children may also mean treating parents. Parents may model anxiety or worry behaviors for children or inadvertently reinforce anxiety statements and behaviors of children (Keeton et al., 2013). Concomitantly, high stress in the family, as well as poor family functioning, can lead to and maintain childhood anxiety disorders (Crawford & Manassis, 2001). Research has indicated that if children experience high levels of stress, additional therapeutic interventions, aimed at decreasing family stress and enhancing child and family coping may be needed to help improve child functioning (e.g., Kiff et al., 2018). Thus, good practice often dictates treatment of the child and working with the parents to reduce anxiety symptoms and change environmental factors that may maintain a child's anxious behaviors. Research shows that child and family influences on child anxiety symptoms are reciprocal, in that both can serve to heighten a child's anxiety (Silverman, Kurtines, Jaccard, & Pina, 2009).

Keeton et al. (2013) examined data from a large treatment trial for childhood anxiety of children and adolescents who had social phobia, Generalized Anxiety Disorder, or separation anxiety. This clinical trial focused on CBT and medication (i.e., sertraline) as treatments for the aforementioned disorders. Findings from this trial indicated that treatments, including CBT, medication, and CBT + medication, were more beneficial than a placebo pill condition. Keeton et al. examined data from the trial to see how parents faired, as the treatments focused on the child. They examined parental distress and anxiety as well as family functioning. Their results indicated that irrespective of type of treatment parental symptoms of distress and anxiety and family functioning improved, but only for children who responded to some type of treatment (i.e., CBT, CBT + sertraline, or sertraline).

Younger Children: Parent–Child Cognitive Behavioral Therapy

Hirschfeld-Becker et al. (2010) conducted a clinical trial to examine the influence of a parent–child CBT intervention for children between the ages of 4–7 years. They enrolled 64 children (53% were girls, mean age was about 5 years) and randomized children to participate in their intervention or a wait-list control group. A strength of this study was that children's symptoms were assessed by interviewers who did not know whether they were assigned to the treatment or wait-list condition. They assessed whether parents had anxiety disorders. Children were enrolled in the study if they had an anxiety disorder, and they were excluded if they experienced psychosis or cognitive delays. If a child was too distractible to participate, then he or she was not enrolled and if a child needed immediate treatment, he or she was referred for services immediately.

Children were randomized to a treatment group, where they received 20 sessions of treatment, or to a wait-list control group (Hirschfeld-Becker et al., 2010). The intervention was conducted by licensed psychologists and one postdoctoral fellow. This intervention was modeled after the Coping Cat Program developed by Kendall (2012). The intervention featured relaxation training, exposure treatment and cognitive restructuring. The activities were restructured for younger children, using games and immediate positive reinforcement for coping attempts and using strategies to manage anxiety. The program for younger children involved parents as trainers, who helped with modeling appropriate behaviors and reinforcing children's coping. This intervention also included parent skills training and treatment for parental anxiety. Results indicated symptom improvement at a 1-year follow-up.

Evidence-Based Strategies: A Literature Review

Silverman, Pina, and Viswesvaran (2008) reviewed 32 studies on treatment of phobias and anxiety disorders. Silverman et al. also reviewed meta-analyses. Of the 32 studies they reviewed, the majority ($n = 22$) featured CBT as the primary treatment.

In the other 10 studies, CBT techniques were used in comparison conditions. Typically, treatment involved 10–15 sessions. They found that several types of CBT interventions (individual, group, and family treatments) were effective for treatment of childhood and adolescent anxiety. However, if group treatment was used, parental involvement or lessons for parents could boost the impact of this treatment. Hence, it may be helpful to have parents observe sessions or review homework (practice strategies) with the child. Manassis et al. (2014) proposed that parent involvement in treatment may be helpful in maintaining effects of treatment, as parents can help with practice. They also can help with rewarding the child. If parents are anxious themselves, they can benefit from learning anxiety management strategies so that they will not be role-modeling anxious responses or inadvertently reinforcing the child's avoidance of anxiety-provoking stimuli/events (Manassis et al., 2014).

Some of the techniques used in previous studies included in vivo or live graded exposures (shaping the child to overcome fear slowly, with reinforcement for success) to a feared stimulus or situation, relaxation training, and reinforcement of positive behaviors (Silverman et al., 2008). A number of studies used different types of CBT, assisting children in managing "upset" emotions, using positive self-talk, and improving family and child communication and problem-solving skills. Others used modeling to help children overcome fear responses. Some studies provided treatment using the Internet, while others used bibliotherapy or manuals to deliver CBT. Practicing strategies, perhaps through role play or social stories where the child can read about different anxiety management strategies helps the child review information and become familiar with using treatment techniques. Silverman and colleagues presented a great review of studies, and although this review was published in 2008, the paper still has significant implications because the studies were well conducted, many with random assignment to groups and wait-list groups. Results were fairly similar to the review by Higa-McMillan et al. (2016), where researchers emphasized exposure to feared stimuli, modeling, and CBT plus medication as being very successful (or top tier) treatments for anxiety. Although exposure has been effective, others have mentioned that further research is needed to determine the mechanisms through which exposure works and that it will be important to determine how exposure is related to long-term outcomes for youth with anxiety (e.g., Peterman, Carper, & Kendall, 2019). In addition, other positive interventions discovered by Higa-McMillan et al. (2016) were relaxation, education, and problem-solving—these interventions were among the second tier of positive interventions for treatment of anxiety.

I will review some of these techniques in the following section of this chapter entitled "Applying Strategies." I have found it beneficial to have children practice the strategies so that they can be used when needed. Moreover, teaching the child to combine strategies and learn what strategies are favorites and can be used routinely is crucial when building the child's repertoire of coping strategies.

Applying Strategies

Explaining the Avoidance Cycle There are many books that are successful in explaining anxiety symptoms and treatments. One reason I believe these books are a helpful tool is that they explain the anxiety cycle in ways that are easy for children to understand. The following explanation exemplifies how I teach children about how avoidance can increase anxiety symptoms. First, anxiety is discussed as being a normal part of life. I mention it is acceptable to have worries, but that they can grow too large. The child and I often draw a picture of the child's anxiety. Then, I draw my own picture of anxiety—a circle with jagged edges and legs, feet, arms, and hands. A face is drawn, with open eyes, a nose and mouth. The figure also has "britches" or pants and shoes. But, anxiety can "grow" and get "too big for its britches or pants." Next, a second picture is drawn, of the figure and jagged edges growing, with an angry face. The figure is described as "too big for its britches (pants)." The next figure shows the "blob" or circle much bigger, "way too large for its britches," with an even larger upset face. I discuss how avoiding and not powering through anxiety causes it to grow and become too big, so the figure is upset and very anxious. The heart of this explanation is that anxiety is "fed" or reinforced by avoidance. I then discuss ways to reset the child's anxiety and system to a lower level, so that the child can power through his or her worries. The importance of natural self-soothing strategies is stressed, and a careful interview with the child can uncover ideas for strategies that the child might be more likely to use, such as distraction, positive imagery, and positive self-talk. The therapist can then help the child practice and learn to use the strategies to assist the child in powering through his or her anxiety.

Negative Self-Talk One of the cognitive components of anxiety that is common in other mental health problems for children is thinking negatively—having a voice inside one's head that talks negatively (negative self-talk such as "I can't do it, I can't go to school, and I can't eat this food"). Helping the child identify negative talk, and learn to use more positive talk and use self-praise can be helpful. I often talk about this negative self-talk as being detrimental to "fun time" and engaging in desired activities because it leads the "listener," if you will, down a negative path that causes avoidance and fear. I also talk with children and adolescents about the fact that bad things are easy to believe, and one needs positive and realistic statements to "talk over" negative voices that speak to you "inside your head."

Children with anxiety may be very performance driven, and want to do things "just right" or perfectly, and this can lead to negative self-evaluation and negative self-talk. Helping the child understand the nature of negative self-talk and the need to be gentler with one's self can be a key component of treatment. In addition, teaching the child to praise his or her efforts and movements toward a goal can be another component of positive self-talk. Furthermore, teaching the child ways to deal with "upsetting emotions" through teaching relaxation, problem-solving skills, and positive self-talk, can provide the child with tools to self-soothe and be calm, thereby lowering physiological arousal which can heighten feelings of anxiety.

Positive self-talk can involve challenging worry and talking back to worry. Many children may believe their anxiety is uncontrollable or "in control" of them. It is important to convince them it is possible to "break into" the anxiety cycle and reduce it or reset one's system in order to face fears and reduce anxiety. It is often necessary to repeat the explanation that avoiding whatever the child is anxious about increases anxiety, feeding anxiety so it grows like a plant. The importance of telling it to "Stop!" or "Shut Up!" is positive or helpful for some children, as it helps to break the "hold" or control they believe anxiety has over them. Some children "psych out" their anxiety saying, "You are not so bad. I am going to win this." Other children may need a superhero they select to talk back to their anxiety so that they can reset and "power through" their anxiety.

Graded Exposure to a Feared Stimulus Another key component of treating many types of anxiety, especially those involving avoidance, is graded exposure. In my practice I have used imaginary and in-vivo graded exposure. For example, Anna, a 10-year-old girl, was afraid of dogs. This fear began when a dog at a pet store bared its teeth and growled at her. When she put her hand to the cage, the dog barked louder and snarled, again bearing its teeth. Anna was very afraid in the pet store. Her mother comforted Anna and quickly removed her from the store. Over a period of 6 months, Anna's fear grew and she became afraid of other dogs. Her fear was so great that she kept her mother from seeing her sister, as their family had a small dog. Although this dog was very friendly, Anna became extremely distraught when her mother mentioned going to see her aunt. When her mother brought Anna for treatment, we all, Anna, her mother and this therapist, agreed she could overcome her fear and get used to being around dogs. We began with looking at pictures of dogs on an iPad. After this, Anna looked at books with pictures of dogs. She had a reward chart, where if she did a good job looking at and touching pictures three times, then she would earn a small treat or get to play a game with her mother.

Anna graduated from books, to YouTube videos of dogs. Then, in a therapy session, Anna, her mother, and I visited a pet store. There was a dog in the doorway, a stroke of luck, because the first goal was to go stand outside a pet store. Anna was very afraid of going in. Nevertheless, Anna did very well with her exposure to the dog (while she was outside). After this, at a next session, we went inside a pet store. While Anna was in a shopping cart, she went past dogs in a cage. We had arranged that there would not be dogs in the aisles we went through. There were dogs behind a glass getting groomed. Anna did well with this exposure. Next, Anna looked at more videos at home. Her mother gave this therapist a call and said that she thought Anna was ready for another step. Her cousin brought the family dog (Anna's aunt's dog) to a therapy session on a Sunday. We had decided to conduct the session when the office was free. The office had a long hallway and Anna began her exposure at the end of the hallway, with lots of praise for facing her fears from Mom and Dad (both wanted to be with Anna as she participated in the exposure session).

After the first exposure in the hallway, the therapist moved Anna a little closer, and Anna did well. The next steps were a surprise. Anna's mother suddenly said, "Anna let's get through this, we miss Aunt Kitty and the family so much." Anna reluctantly agreed to go closer. Her mother mentioned to Anna that she used to be such good friends with her cousin's dog. Her cousin encouraged Anna to pet the dog and she did. Anna was very pleased with herself. She petted the dog several times and went home. Next, Anna's mother took her to see her sister and Anna petted the dog some more, for brief periods. Then, a birthday party came, and Anna went to her aunt's home. The dog came out during the party—and this encounter was successful. Soon after this, Anna and her family were able to visit her aunt's house and her mother said the treatment was successful. Not all sessions go this well. There are many with stumbling blocks and periods where there is not progress. This case was presented as an example of a graded exposure technique that began with a reinforcement (reward) chart, moved to praise of the positive behavior, and then rewards were withdrawn as the child was very proud of her progress and very happy to be able to interact with her aunt's dog again.

Santucci, Thomassin, Petrovic, and Weisz (2015) proposed that exposure to a feared stimulus was an essential part of treatment. They recommended use of different strategies, such as relaxation and distraction, to help the child manage the physiological symptoms related to anxious thinking. When changing the child's negative cognitions or beliefs that he or she cannot control anxiety, it can be beneficial to help the child think about his or her problem differently—as something that can be overcome. Moreover, in order for the child to easily access the strategies, therapists may provide homework, as suggested by Kendall (2012), so that coping strategies are more readily accessible and familiar to the child when anxious thinking and physiological symptoms occur. The child should practice and even over-learn strategies as a relapse prevention strategy. Predicting that anxiety will recur or that the child will feel nervous and need to apply strategies in the future may be essential even after anxiety has decreased or abated, as anxious symptoms and situations can recur or take different avenues as the child develops.

Relaxation and Distraction Several other techniques, briefly mentioned by Silverman et al. (2008) can be helpful therapeutic tools. Relaxation, through breathing and muscle relaxation, can help "reset" the child's system, and lower heart rate, breathing and muscle tension, so that the child is in a more relaxed state to power through his or her anxiety. I believe that resetting physiologically can be helpful for children who are experiencing anxiety. A reset in the middle of a child's anxiety cycle also may help a child to interrupt repetitive thoughts that result in anxiety and further reduce his or her physiological arousal. Breathing and muscle relaxation can work differently in young children. Children may not be able to engage in extended periods of deep breathing or traditional progressive muscle relaxation strategies. For breathing, I teach the child to fill up his or her stomach with air. In order to help with breathing in through the child's nose, I instruct the child to "smell a flower." Then, the child holds his or her breath for a count of three to five. This is to stop shallow breathing. After this, the child is taught to release the breath slowly, by a count of three. If the child has difficulty slowly releasing his or her breath, then I work with the child to practice slowly blowing out the birthday candles on a cake.

Children may have difficulty with progressive muscle relaxation. It may be hard for them to move from larger (e.g., shoulder area) to smaller muscle areas (e.g., hands and fingers). They might not have the patience to slowly relax. I often have children use a rock and sponge technique. The child makes his or her body hard like a rock for a count of three to five and then becomes a sponge for a "long time," which is a count of 30 or more seconds. If children count too fast, they can put their name in between a number such as, "… one, Molly, two Molly, three Molly, four Molly, and five Molly." I typically role model for the child, practicing breathing and muscle relaxation, and then discuss the importance of practicing the techniques at home. The parent also observes the practice, so that he or she can assist the child in practicing the techniques at home and administer rewards for successful management of symptoms of anxiety (Manassis et al., 2014).

Distraction can involve doing something fun, like playing a song or doing a puzzle. Some children watch a calming video on their iPad, or they close their eyes and listen to a short calming video, such as those that feature waves hitting against the sand or rain. Others benefit from reading a book or talking things through with a trusted adult. Distraction can be a key component in a "reset" process. After a brief reset break, powering through the anxiety, so it does not grow too large is stressed. Tailoring the distraction strategy to the child's own experiences and personality is key. Using positive mental imagery can be a form of mental distraction for some children. For instance, one child I worked with had anxiety-related migraines. He developed the image of the "Incredible Hulk" wielding his hammer to "hammer out" problems and pain related to his headache. Imagining the Hulk distracted him from repetitive thoughts and was a positive strategy he could use whenever he become anxious at school.

Dialing Down Worry and Anxiety Another idea that has been helpful for some children is to "dial down" the anxiety. This involves learning about anxiety triggers, how anxiety grows (often using a thermometer or meter), and ways to decrease anxiety so that it is not debilitating. The child can employ a variety of strategies to decrease symptoms of anxiety, after identifying that it is growing too large or increasing in intensity to an unacceptable level.

For this strategy, children can learn about the anxiety cycle and how it increases on the anxiety meter until it grows too big (i.e., too high) and the anxiety meter is overwhelmed. The anxiety meter is a thermometer that shows how anxiety can grow. Next, the child can keep notes or a diary to learn about his or her anxiety triggers. Another way to learn about triggers—or events that begin anxiety symptoms--is to complete a diary or notes within a therapy session with the help of the child and parents. This is helpful if they can not take notes about what happens at home and in other settings. It is valuable to ensure that the child also learns reset strategies that he or she can apply when his or her anxiety is triggered and the worry cycle begins. The therapist can explain to the child that it is beneficial to catch anxiety when it is first triggered or early in the worry phase, so that the reset strategies can be used to bring it down to size or alleviate it. The reset strategies, such as breathing, relaxing, and challenge (i.e., challenging the worry thoughts to stop), can help the child move the anxiety meter downward, in order to face or power through things he or she is worried about. If the reset strategies are practiced earlier in the cycle of growth, then the anxiety can be reduced earlier, and the child can either power through the anxiety-provoking event or problem-solve and decide how to resolve an anxiety-provoking situation.

Personalizing Anxiety Management Strategies I have made a coping book with the child that features strategies, written in a developmentally appropriate way, that the child can read at home. The coping book contains the child's preferred anxiety management strategies, such as relaxation, imagery, distraction, challenging anxious thoughts, or using logic to understand if the anxiety provoking thoughts are true. Before making a book, I explain how the strategies work. Then, the child and I practice using the strategies and record them in the child's book, with the child drawing illustrations to personalize and decorate his or her book.

For other children, a therapist can make a coping menu (Nabors, Stough, Combs, & Elkins, 2019). For the coping menu, the child picks the name of his or her restaurant. Then, the child selects coping strategies for the menu. The first type of strategy is relaxation. This therapist writes down relaxation strategies, such as listening to a relaxing video, breathing, or muscle relaxation. Specifics are recorded, such as how many breaths to take and how long the child will be a rock (3–5 s) and how long the child will be a sponge (30 or more seconds). The next area on the menu is imagery. If a superhero is chosen, the name of this hero is recorded on the menu. The child is also taught to go to (or imagine) his or her favorite place or event, which can be an amusement park, the beach, a birthday party, and so on. The therapist teaches the child to imagine this happy event or time in detail, recalling sights, smells, sounds, and other details. For instance, if the child is walking on the beach, then he or she should hear the waves and birds, feel the sand underfoot, pick up a shell, and then feel the waves on his or her feet after he or she runs into the water and runs back. When personalizing strategies, the child can select imagery that is very active, such as watching fireworks or going to an amusement park. The key is finding something that is relaxing, distracting, and fun for the child. Then, teaching the child to imagine things like he or she is "in a movie" may help the child visualize a scene or event. At times, a child has imagined him or herself inside a favorite movie or television show, such as one child who imagined himself as "Harry Potter at Hogwarts." Other strategies may be listed on the child's menu (e.g., doing something fun, getting support from parents, using challenge words to "talk back" to worries).

Worry Detective (Using Problem-Solving) Another way to help a child personalize strategies is to introduce the concept of being a "worry detective" (Kendall, 2012). The therapist can teach the child that worries are sneaky and to learn to spot them and then apply different strategies or combinations of strategies to reduce worries. For example, some children may be "distractors" and need to apply one or more distraction strategies, like doing something fun or thinking of his or her "happy place" to stop a worry from growing. Another child may need to reset and "dial down" a worry so that he or she can go through it, such as a child who needs to relax and learn to enjoy being in the choir and performing in front of others. This child may benefit from breathing and using "rock-sponge" and then powering through by going on stage. If a child is having a "hard" worry day, with lots of anxiety, it may take several strategies and attempts to work through anxiety. As a worry detective, the child needs to catch himself or herself worrying before the worry grows, and then decide what strategy or strategies to apply. The child needs to problem-solve to decide which strategies to use and how often.

Desensitization Primeau et al. (2016) wrote that systematic desensitization "… is based on the principle of reciprocal inhibition in which the individual is taught to apply a relaxing response when presented with an anxiety-provoking stimuli." (p. 359). The systematic desensitization requires graded exposure, with the child being relaxed as he or she successfully masters each level of exposure. Let us again use the example of wanting to avoid performing in front of others, due to anxiety. Prior to the concert, the therapist could use graded exposure, with the child practicing being relaxed and on stage, with his or her parents as an audience. This practice can also occur "in vivo" or through imagination where the therapist has the child write out his or her fears about performing on notecards, orders them in the order of fearfulness (e.g., an anxiety hierarchy), and then the therapist helps the child imagine going through each scene while the child is relaxed. Children should order cards from least fearful to most fearful and the therapist can begin with the "least" fearful card, help the child relax and move through the situation in his or her imagination while relaxed, and then try another harder card. The therapist may not get through all the cards in one session, but should stop on a card that the child has successfully mastered by relaxing through the situation in his or her imagination. This type of "graded exposure" mirrors a systematic desensitization process (Ollendick & King, 1998).

Social Skills Silverman et al. (2008) also mentioned teaching social skills and improving the child's social network as possible treatment components for some children. This may be valuable for children with Social Anxiety Disorder (SAD). Spence and Rapee (2015) proposed that an interplay of individual and environmental variables influences the development of SAD, such that there are several pathways (combinations of factors) that can result in the development of this disorder. Hence, taking a careful history and changing both the child's environment and enhancing skill sets can be components of treatment.

For children with SAD, avoidance of social situations may have caused skills deficits. Conversely, it may be that a lack of social skills enhances social anxiety. Teaching friendship skills, such as how to enter a group, invite others to play, how to ask for help and assistance, and how to carry on a conversation may be helpful tools for children with social fears. Children with social phobia also may use graded exposures in a variety of situations to gain social experience. Reinforcement for going to birthday parties, going to sports events and practices, and performing in front of others may be needed, in addition to teaching relaxation and social skills, to help children with social anxiety face and begin to participate in different social experiences. Hoffman and Otto (2017) offer a great text, highlighting evidence-based treatments for social anxiety disorder, entitled, "*Cognitive Behavioral Therapy for Social Anxiety Disorder: Evidence-Based and Disorder Specific Treatment Techniques*." This book features case examples and also provides information on medications, and can serve as a useful guide for clinicians treating clients with SAD.

Reviewing What Works

Higa-McMillan et al. (2016) wrote a more recent review to update the evidence base on treatment of anxiety in children and adolescents. They commented that although there is a lot of information available, it may be difficult to access recent information on effective treatments. Their review included 111 clinical trials with over 200 treatment conditions. They also utilized a practice profile to depict types of practices used for specific problems. They used a classification system, which helped separate treatments. For instance, they classified exposure and other types of CBT separately. They reported that exposure treatments, without CBT components, were effective in treatment of anxiety. This is encouraging because it implies that "grandma's cure" or "facing the fear and powering through anxiety" can be effective. This type of treatment may, at times, be quick and effective in helping children overcome anxiety. However, it is noteworthy that CBT treatments that were combined with exposure therapy had large effect sizes. Using exposure with other techniques may enhance its impact. Similar to Silverman et al. (2008), Higa-McMillan et al. concluded that both individual and group treatments had effective results in treatment of anxiety. Higa-McMillan et al. reviewed family, Internet-based, and combination formats for delivering treatments and found that these treatments could be effective.

Higa-McMillan et al. (2016) reported that exposure was the most common practice element used in treatment, used over 80% of the time. One example of a successful exposure program is the Child Anxiety Multi-Day Program or CAMP for children who experience separation anxiety (Santucci & Ehrenreich-May, 2013). This program begins as a day camp for children and they are involved in a series of activities. The day camp ends with a therapeutic sleepover. This program has been successful and is an example of outside the box thinking and real-life exposure that can improve separation anxiety. Higa-McMillan et al. (2016) proposed that cognitive techniques, such as using positive self- talk, were used just over 60% of the time and this was followed by relaxation techniques used a little over 50% of the time. Many of the treatments included educational components to teach children, or children and their parents, about the influence of anxiety on the child, triggers for anxiety, and how anxiety affects the body. These treatment techniques were followed by modeling (showing a child how to overcome fear) and reward—labeled as self-reward or self-praise. I use self-praise with children and have them monitor their progress on a reward chart. On the other hand, I also involve parents in providing rewards, especially at the initiation of treatment, as in the case of Anna. It is often the case that small rewards are replaced by praise and fall away as the child experiences success. The reward charts fade at different rates, depending on the child's characteristics, parents' use of the reward system, and the result of environmental exposures (whether they are successful, the amount of effort needed from the child, etc.; Manassis et al., 2014).

When I work with younger children, the parent or parents often accompany the child to therapy sessions, and we make an anxiety management book, filled with strategies that work for the child, and the child and parent practice these strategies together (as homework). Their practice or homework assignment is to review the strategies for a week by reading the child's coping book or coping menu each day. The child may apply strategies, while engaging in practice with strategies while reviewing the book. Even if the strategies are not used, children may benefit from reviewing and practicing the strategies to learn new skills. The parent is involved in treatment, and many parents report benefitting from practicing with their child. Often, they sheepishly admit, as therapy progresses, that they experience anxiety (Manassis et al., 2014). Higa-McMillan et al. (2016) pointed out that anxious self-talk, which I earlier termed as negative self-talk, can mediate treatment outcome. Moreover, when providing therapy, I may encourage replacing negative self-talk with positive words. I can encourage the child to use positive images, such as a child's own superhero to fight negative words and images. Higa-McMillan et al. did find a study showing that rewards help the child when working through exposures, which was definitely the case at the outset of Anna's treatment to overcome her phobia related to dogs.

It was evident that the literature was expanding and meeting the goals set by Silverman et al. (2008), as Higa-McMillan et al. (2016) were able to examine the impact of mediators and moderators of successful anxiety treatments. For example, they indicated children with more severe baseline pathology or whose parents are experiencing mental health disorders may be less likely to benefit from CBT. Similar to Silverman et al. (2008), Higa-McMillan et al. found that girls and younger children have more positive responses to use of CBT techniques and family involvement in treatment. Higa-McMillan et al. (2016) found that exposure and CBT remained effective treatments, which is consistent with findings by Silverman et al. (2008). Higa-McMillan et al. recommended that for many childhood anxiety problems, this literature—exposure and CBT—was a starting point and that clinicians should search this literature and find evidence-based treatments that apply to the case they are treating. CBT combined with anxiety decreasing medications were also effective, top tier treatments (Higa-McMillan et al., 2016).

Where to Go in the Future Higa-McMillan et al. (2016) mentioned that we need to learn more about the durability of treatment. I would agree with this. We need to learn how many children return for treatment, after they finish a round of treatment?

How many children require treatment again, require booster sessions, or require treatment in adulthood? We also need to learn more about comorbid conditions, as many children with anxiety present with other mental health problems, which can have a long-term impact on their social and emotional development (Whiteside et al., 2016). The purpose of this book is to improve understanding of comorbid conditions, from a clinical frame with case examples, in the hopes of spurring further research to improve our knowledge of treating comorbid conditions in children and adolescents. Silverman et al. (2008) called for more research with children from low-income families and children from minority groups. Kendall et al. (2016) similarly called for further research on treatment of anxiety for youth residing in minority groups. Silverman et al. (2008) noted research focusing on children who did not complete treatment will expand knowledge about the impact of anxiety treatments, and I believe that this call for studies is helpful today. Moreover, delivering treatment in new ways, to reach many children, using Internet-based protocols, may improve access to evidence-based techniques.

Translating the Evidence Base Using Critical "Modules" or Aspects of EBTs

Kendall's (2012) program has been very effective in treatment of anxiety and parts of his training have generalized to being included in modular treatment experiences. A modular approach uses treatment processes and techniques from evidence-based treatments to treat many different types of psychiatric problems (Santucci et al., 2015). Weisz et al. (2012) support the use of treatment modules, or effective cognitive behavioral treatments, which can be used to treat different symptoms associated with child anxiety, depression, trauma, and conduct problems. A flowchart can be used to determine which treatment technique to use with different symptoms for different types of mental health problems (Santucci et al., 2015). A flowchart may assist the therapist in determining which treatments work for comorbid problems. This has the potential to shorten treatment and make it less complex.

I believe that therapists need to move between components of effective practice in order to treat children with comorbid conditions, and that the cognitive-behavioral treatments allow such movement. Park, Chorpita, Regan, and Weisz (2014) found that youth who participated in modular treatment received treatment in fewer different mental health settings after a year. In another study, Chorpita et al. (2017) demonstrated that modular treatment can be flexible and using modular therapy could result in faster gains in symptom reduction compared to community-based treatments. This may occur because the modular approach makes it easier to address multiple problems and symptoms with similar treatments. Weisz and colleagues have been working to bridge the gap between clinical trials research and real-world clinical practice (e.g., Weisz, Sandler, Durlak, & Anton, 2006). The STEPs Program—or the Child System and Treatment Enhancement Projects—uses treatment ideas from evidence-based practice to treat a variety of psychological problems in children (Schoenwald, Kelleher, & Weisz, 2008).

Kendall and his colleagues suggested that "… a stepped care approach accounts for the fact that not all youth experiencing interfering anxiety need the same level of care" (p. 1). Some children will require a longer course of treatment, using many strategies, and for these children, anxiety may take different forms, such as separation anxiety that transfers to a fear of group performances at school. Monitoring the impact of interventions and the child's anxiety level can provide critical data. Thus, understanding what (which treatment strategies) decreases anxiety and how much anxiety decreases is central to monitoring the influence of treatment. Using bibliotherapy to shorten the length of treatment, websites with helpful information, and other short-term treatments are a great first step in treatment. Then, after checking the success of the treatment, the therapist can determine whether more intensive intervention is necessary. Group and individual treatments can be effective (e.g., Silverman et al., 2008) and pharmacotherapy may be an option for some children (Kendall et al., 2016). In deciding whether to "step up" treatment several other factors, including family functioning, parent anxiety, children's success with initial treatments, and comorbid conditions for the child should be considered (Kendall et al., 2016). If the child therapist remains within a family framework and considers the individual child's situation and personality characteristics, he or she can develop a tailored, individualized treatment program that will assist the child in coping with multiple psychological problems.

I believe that the notion of personalizing treatment to meet children where they are, and tailoring the intervention to "fit" their situation and personalities will allow therapists to translate information in the evidence base to help children (Santucci et al., 2015). I believe that Santucci et al.'s ideas for thinking about how to use interventions in the field when developing evidence-based programs are critical. Doing this may help ensure transportability of interventions to "everyday" or "regular" clinical practice. Furthermore, ensuring that practitioners have a role in designing and implementing clinical trials and treatments is another way to potentially improve transportability (Santucci et al., 2015). I think that clinicians would agree with Santucci et al. that "noise" or things that happen over the course of treatment impact the effectiveness of one's interventions and the next steps the clinician takes.

Brief Case Description

The following description is of a case that identified "noise"—parents going on a vacation and a coincidental child illness—as key determinants of a relapse into anxiety symptoms. Sally was an adolescent who experienced school refusal. She had attended three sessions and had confronted her fears. She had used breathing and listening to music to overcome school anxiety and school refusal. After her second successful week of attending school, her parents went on vacation in Europe. She was being watched by her great aunt. Part of her symptoms was stomach upset related to her anxiety. Soon after her parents left, as luck would have it, Sally got a stomach bug. She did try to go to school and had an upset stomach and was sent home by the school nurse. The flu-like symptoms had Sally throwing up and experiencing stomach upset the first week her parents were away. During the second week of their vacation, when Sally was set to return to school, she reexperienced her anxiety symptoms. She hid under the bed, which was her previous coping strategy. She refused to go to school due to anxiety and her stomach feeling upset. Sally was again worried that she would become sick at school. She stayed out of school for another week, with her schoolwork piling up and increasing anxiety symptoms.

Her parents returned to, as her mother described it, "a crisis." This was a "mountain of homework" that Sally would not complete and thus a full return of anxiety symptoms. Moreover, Sally refused to return to counseling or therapy, hiding under her bed so her mother could not bring her to her appointment. She would not follow any recommendations for treatment. Lack of adherence to treatment recommendations can be a barrier to the success of anxiety management interventions (Lee et al., 2019). Now, the "noise" of her parents leaving sparked some separation issues, which were related to her anxiety over school. Her mother's tendency to describe and react to issues in a "crisis mode" exacerbated the situation. This noise and individual characteristics are crucial to explaining this case. This type of information might be glossed over in a clinical trial, or this child would have been considered either a treatment success or failure depending upon when surveys were completed and according to what was defined as an endpoint of treatment. Unfortunately, this case had several complications, which could be critical in determining outcomes in a private practice setting.

In terms of working with the school, the therapist initially contacted teachers—the two that were providing homework that was overwhelming to Sally. She arranged for them to speak with Sally and coach her about ways to be successful in completing her work. The therapist contacted the principal, who worked closely with students. She described Sally's issues and the principal arranged for Sally to be able to come to the office and speak with her for a moment, if she was feeling anxious. The principal talked with Sally about how valuable she was to the school, both as a student and as a "cheerleader," who was always supportive of her classmates. Having a special place to discuss her troubles was a "boost" for Sally's self-esteem. The teachers, too, were supportive. They did not reduce the workload, but allowed Sally extra time to complete work. They allowed her extra time on tests. If needed, the school counselor (there was not a school psychologist) and teachers agreed to meet to develop a special plan to assist with providing extra time and support on tests and homework if Sally needed this. They recommended a special plan be developed rather than a Section 504 Plan as it was a private school. However, in public schools, Section 504 plans can be helpful, providing structure and guidelines that can follow a child at different grade levels.

Conclusions

This chapter reviews the importance of using evidence-based strategies in a strategic manner, in order to help children manage their anxiety (e.g., Higa-McMillan et al., 2016; Silverman et al., 2008). Parent involvement can be beneficial when the child needs rewards for working on graded exposure to a feared stimulus or when the parent also has anxiety. Parent involvement can, in some cases, extend the value of treatment over the maintenance phase as well (Manassis et al., 2014). Strategies to use with children include positive self-talk, desensitization, graded exposure, distraction, relaxation, positive imagery, and muscle relaxation (Silverman et al., 2008). Homework sessions that allow the child to learn strategies so that they become routine can be helpful. Teaching the child to apply a variety of strategies in combination when anxiety symptoms are strong may help the child power through his or her anxiety. Anxiety can co-occur with other mental health problems. As such, a modular approach (Park et al., 2014), where the therapist selects strategies that may be effective for anxiety and other mental health issues, may help the child experience a shorter course of treatment. In the future, more research on nonadherence to interventions will provide useful information for clinicians (Lee et al., 2019) as will research on variables associated with specific treatments that are related to decreases in anxiety.

References

Caron, C., & Rutter, M. (1991). Comorbidity in child psychopathology: Concepts, issues, and research strategies. *Journal of Child Psychology & Psychiatry & Allied Disciplines, 32*(7), 1063–1080. https://doi.org/10.1111/j1469-7610.1991.tb00350x

Chorpita, B. F., Daleiden, E. L., Park, A. L., Ward, A. M., Levy, M. C., Cromley, T., … Krull, J. L. (2017). Child STEPs in California: A cluster randomized effectiveness trial comparing modular treatment with community implemented treatment for youth with anxiety, depression, conduct problems, or traumatic stress. *Journal of Consulting and Clinical Psychology, 85*(1), 13–25. https://doi.org/10.1037/ccp0000133

Crawford, A. M., & Manassis, K. (2001). Familial predictors of treatment outcome in childhood anxiety disorders. *Journal of the American Academy of Child and Adolescent Psychiatry, 40*, 1182–1189. https://doi.org/10.1097/00004583-200110000-00012

Higa-McMillan, C. K., Francis, S. E., Rith-Najarian, L., & Chorpita, B. F. (2016). Evidence-base update: 50 years of research on treatment for child and adolescent anxiety. *Journal of Clinical Child and Adolescent Psychology, 45*(2), 91–113. https://doi.org/10.1080/15374416.2015.1046177

Hirschfeld-Becker, D. R., Dina, R., Masek, B., Henin, A., Blakely, L. R., Pollock-Wurman, R. A., … Biederman, J. (2010). Cognitive-behavioral therapy for 4- to 7-year-old children with anxiety disorders: A randomized clinical trial. *Journal of Consulting and Clinical Psychology, 78*(4), 498–510. https://doi.org/10.1037/a0019055

Hoffman, S. G., & Otto, M. W. (2017). *Cognitive behavioral therapy for social anxiety disorder: Evidence-based and disorder specific treatment techniques* (2nd ed.). New York: Routledge.

Keeton, C. P., Ginsburg, G. S., Drake, K. L., Sakolsky, D., Kendall, P. C., Birmaher, B., … Walkup, J. T. (2013). Benefits of child-focused anxiety treatments for parents and family functioning. *Depression and Anxiety, 30*(9), 865–872. https://doi.org/10.1002/da.22055

Kendall, P. C. (2012). Anxiety disorders in youth. In P. C. Kendall (Ed.), *Child and adolescent therapy: Cognitive-behavioral procedures* (4th ed., pp. 143–189). New York: Guilford Press.

Kendall, P. C., Gosch, E., Furr, J. M., & Sood, E. (2008). Flexibility within fidelity. *Journal of the American Academy of Child and Adolescent Psychiatry, 47*, 987–993. https://doi.org/10.1097/CHI.0b013e31817eed2f

Kendall, P. C., & Hedtke, K. A. (2006a). *Cognitive behavioral therapy for anxious children: Therapist manual 3*. Ardmore, PA: Workbook Publishing.

Kendall, P. C., & Hedtke, K. A. (2006b). *Coping cat workbook 2*. Ardmore, PA: Workbook Publishing.

Kendall, P. C., Makover, H., Swan, A., Carper, M. M., Mercado, R., Kagan, E., & Crawford, E. (2016). What steps to take? How to approach concerning anxiety in youth. *Clinical Psychology: Science and Practice, 23*(3), 211–229. https://doi.org/10.1111/cpsp.12156

Kiff, C. J., Ernestus, S., Gonzalez, A., Kendall, P. C., Albano, A. M., Compton, S. N., … Piacentini, J. (2018). The interplay of familial and individual risk in predicting clinical improvements in pediatric anxiety disorders. *Journal of Clinical Child & Adolescent Psychology, 47*(S1), S542–S554. https://doi.org/10.1080/15374416.2018.1460848

Lee, P., Zehgeer, A., Ginsburg, G., McCracken, J., Keeton, C., Kendall, P. C., … Compton, S. (2019). Child and adolescent adherence with cognitive behavioral therapy for anxiety: Predictors and associations with outcomes. *Journal of Clinical Child & Adolescent Psychology, 48*(S1), S215–S226. https://doi.org/10.1080/15374416.2017.1310046

Manassis, K., Lee, T. C., Bennett, K., Zhao, X. Y., Mendlowitz, S., Duda, S., … Wood, J. J. (2014). Types of parental involvement in CBT with anxious youth: A preliminary meta-analysis. *Journal of Consulting and Clinical Psychology, 82*(6), 1163–1172. https://doi.org/10.1037/a0036969

Nabors, L., Odar Stough, C., Combs, A., & Elkins, J. (2019). Implementing the *coping positively with my worries manual*: A pilot study. *Journal of Child and Family Studies, 28*(10), 2708–2717. https://doi.org/10.1007/s10826-019-01451-3

Ollendick, T. H., & King, N. J. (1998). Empirically supported treatments for children with phobic and anxiety disorders: Current status. *Journal of Clinical Child Psychology, 27*(2), 156–167. https://doi.org/10.1207/s15374424jccp2702_3

Öst, L.-G., & Ollendick, T. H. (2017). Brief, intensive and concentrated cognitive behavioral treatments for anxiety disorders in children: A systematic review and meta-analysis. *Behaviour Research and Therapy, 97*, 134–145. https://doi.org/10.1016/j.brat.2017.07.008

Park, A. L., Chorpita, B. F., Regan, J., & Weisz, J. R. (2014). Integrity of evidence-based practice: Are providers modifying practice content or practice sequencing? *Administration and Policy in Mental Health and Mental Health Services Research, 42*(2), 186–196. https://doi.org/10.1007/s10488-014-0559-z

Peterman, J. S., Carper, M. M., & Kendall, P. C. (2019). Testing the habituation-based model of exposures for child and adolescent anxiety. *Journal of Child & Adolescent Psychology, 48*(S1), S34–S44. https://doi.org/10.1080/15374416.2016.1163707

Piacentini, J., Bennett, S., Compton, S. N., Kendall, P. C., Birmaher, B., Albano, A. M., … Walkup, J. (2014). 24- and 36-week outcomes for the child/adolescent anxiety multimodal study (CAMS). *Journal of the American Academy of Child & Adolescent Psychiatry, 53*(3), 297–310. https://doi.org/10.1016/j.jaac.2013.11.010

Primeau, M., Gershon, A., Talbot, L., Cotto, I., Lotspeich, L., Hardan, A., … O'Hara, R. (2016). Individuals with autism spectrum disorders have equal success rate but require longer periods of systematic desensitization than control patients to complete ambulatory polysomnography. *Journal of Clinical Sleep Medicine, 12*(3), 357–362. https://doi.org/10.5664/jcsm.5584

Santucci, L., & Ehrenreich-May, J. (2013). A randomized controlled trail of the child anxiety multi-day program (CAMP) for separation anxiety disorder. *Child Psychiatry and Human Development, 44*, 439–451. https://doi.org/10.1007/s10578-012-0338-6

Santucci, L. C., Thomassin, K., Petrovic, L., & Weisz, J. R. (2015). Building evidence-based interventions for the youth, providers, and contexts of real-world mental health care. *Child Development Perspectives, 9*(2), 67–73. https://doi.org/10.1111/cdep.12118

Schoenwald, S. K., Kelleher, K., & Weisz, J. (2008). Building bridges to evidence-based practice: The MacArthur Foundation child system and treatment enhancement projects (Child STEPs). *Administration and Policy in Mental Health and Mental Health Services Research, 35*(1–2), 66–72. https://doi.org/10.1007/s10488-007-0160-9

Silverman, W. K., Kurtines, W. M., Jaccard, J., & Pina, A. A. (2009). Directionality of change in youth anxiety treatment involving parents: An initial examination. *Journal of Consulting and Clinical Psychology, 77*, 474–485. https://doi.org/10.1037/a0015761

Silverman, W. K., Pina, A. A., & Viswesvaran, C. (2008). Evidence-based psychosocial treatments for phobic and anxiety disorders in children and adolescents. *Clinical Child and Adolescent Psychology, 37*(1), 105–130. https://doi.org/10.1080/15374410701817907

Silverman, W. K., & Treffers, P. D. (Eds.). (2001). *Anxiety disorders in children and adolescents: Research, assessment and intervention* (pp. 313–334). New York, NY: Cambridge University Press.

Spence, S. H., & Rapee, R. M. (2015). The etiology of social anxiety disorder: An evidence-based model. *Behaviour Research and Therapy, 86*, 50–67. https://doi.org/10.1016/j.brat.2016.06.007

Walkup, J., Albano, A. M., Piacentini, J., Birmaher, B., Compton, S. N., Sherrill, J. T., … March, J. S. (2008). Cognitive behavioral therapy, sertraline, and their combination for children and adolescents with anxiety disorders: Acute phase efficacy and safety. *New England Journal of Medicine, 359*, 2753–2766. https://doi.org/10.1056/NEJMoa0804633

Weisz, J. R., Chorpita, B. F., Palinkas, L. A., Schoenwald, S. K., Miranda, J., Bearman, S. K., … the Research Network on Youth Mental Health. (2012). Testing standard and modular designs for psychotherapy treating depression, anxiety, and conduct problems in youth: A randomized effectiveness trial. *Archives of General Psychiatry, 69*, 274–282. https://doi.org/10.1001/archgenpsychiatry.2011.147

Weisz, J. R., Sandler, I. N., Durlak, J. A., & Anton, B. S. (2006). A proposal to unite two different worlds of children's mental health. *American Psychologist, 61*, 644–645. https://doi.org/10.1037/0003-066X.61.6.644

Whiteside, S. P. H., Deacon, B. J., Benito, K., & Stewart, E. (2016). Factors associated with practitioners' use of exposure therapy for childhood anxiety disorders. *Journal of Anxiety Disorders, 40*, 29–36. https://doi.org/10.1016/janxdis.2016.04.001

Chapter 3
Depression and Anxiety in Children

Introduction

Anxiety and depression commonly co-occur in children and adolescents (Cohen, Young, Gibb, Hankin, & Abela, 2014; Kertz, Sylvester, Tillman, & Luby, 2018). Youth with anxiety who tend to ruminate about worries and be self-critical may be more likely to experience depression if the aforementioned symptoms persist over time (Cohen et al., 2014). Avoidance of social interactions and consistently blaming oneself for one's flaws may contribute to the onset of depression (Cohen et al., 2014). Children with anxiety, who also have significant depression and experience high levels of stress (e.g., adversity), may be at risk for chronic symptoms of anxiety and depression (e.g., Kertz et al., 2018). Experiencing anxiety and depression is related to elevated risk for suicide attempts, higher levels of social anxiety, and poorer child and family functioning (Cummings, Caporino, & Kendall, 2014). Anxiety and depression can be precursors to substance use and suicide in children (Martinsen, Kendall, Stark, & Neumer, 2016). Therefore, treatment of both mental health problems is important to ensure positive emotional development of children. Additionally, Wolk, Beidas, and Kendall (2015) assessed adults who had received treatment as children. They found that participating in therapy was associated with long-term benefits, including protection from suicidal ideation.

Chu and Harrison (2007) conducted a meta-analysis to detect mediators of change in youth with anxiety and depression. They noted overlapping features of treatment, such as identification of thinking errors (i.e., cognitive distortions), the need for developing "coping-oriented" thinking, gaining exposure to pleasurable events, and gaining skills for successfully completing difficult tasks. Further, Chu and Harrison (2007) described reducing fear responses and decreasing avoidance as key behavioral strategies for treating anxiety. They discussed behavioral activation strategies for depression, involving "activating behaviors" to overcome withdrawal and increase the client's involvement in pleasurable activities and social interactions.

L. Nabors, *Anxiety Management in Children with Mental and Physical Health Problems*, Springer Series on Child and Family Studies,
https://doi.org/10.1007/978-3-030-35606-4_3

They highlighted that avoidance, such as withdrawal from social activities, is a key feature of depression. Hence, increasing exposure to social activities was a key treatment for depression. Developing a more positive conceptualization of the self could improve symptoms of anxiety and depression. Finally, they emphasized using a functional assessment (identifying triggers, behavior, and what reinforces the behavior or the consequences of the behavior) to understand what triggered responses and maintained them. They did note different processes were effective in treating anxiety and depression. The cognitive-behavioral therapy (CBT) techniques were more effective for anxiety than depression. The CBT interventions, however, were still somewhat effective in changing thinking patterns for youth who were experiencing depression.

Cummings et al. (2014) proposed three pathways with anxiety occurring prior to depression, both anxiety and depression occurring at the same time, and with depression predating anxiety. If anxiety is the primary condition, then it should be a focus of treatment. Similarly, if depression is the primary diagnosis, then this should be the focus of treatment. If both problems co-occur, or are operating simultaneously, then a transdiagnostic approach, treating both conditions, may be warranted (Ehrenreich-May & Chu, 2014). This may be beneficial for younger children where anxiety and depression often occur as a unitary construct, which is united by a negative emotional responding and believing negative things will occur (Garber & Weersing, 2010). Garber and Weersing (2010) recommended using a combined treatment approach that involves lessons to reduce negative thinking and to reduce avoidance of negative emotions. They encouraged using graded engagement in problem-solving to detect and change negative emotions and increase positive responses to stress.

Prevalence

Both depression and anxiety occur within families, presupposing a genetic predisposition to internalizing problems (Garber & Weersing, 2010). The comorbidity varies from 15 to 75%—with higher rates occurring in clinical samples (Cummings et al., 2014; Garber & Weersing, 2010). Anxiety and depression may be more common in girls than boys (Cummings et al., 2014). Both depression and anxiety can be either chronic or recurring (Werner-Seidler, Perry, Calear, Newby, & Christensen, 2017). Garber and Weersing (2010) wrote that

> The prognosis for comorbid anxiety and depression is worse than either condition alone, with higher risk of recurrence, longer duration, increased suicide attempts, greater impairment, less favorable responses to treatment, and greater utilization of mental health services. (p. 293)

In general, during childhood anxiety predates depression (Garber & Weersing, 2010). Symptoms of depression vary by type of anxiety disorder, although children with anxiety and symptoms of distress are more likely to be depressed (Cummings et al., 2014).

Transdiagnostic Approach

Yap, Pilkington, and Ryan (2014) conducted a literature review of 24 articles examining parental factors associated with anxiety and depression, 140 articles examining parental factors associated with depression, and 17 examining parental factors associated with anxiety. Yap et al. (2014) supported a transdiagnostic approach to treatment. A transdiagnostic approach, implementing positive treatments for multiple symptoms, may be a good way to treat anxiety and depression. The reason for this is that there are many pathways to developing comorbid symptoms and many different trajectories that symptoms can take (Cummings et al., 2014). Yap et al. (2014) recommended that prevention and treatment programs target the following parent behaviors: aversive behaviors, interparental conflict, and overinvolvement by parents. Improving parental warmth was also deemed significant. Yap et al. (2014) did state that overinvolvement of parents may be more commonly associated with anxiety; but, it may be associated with depressive symptoms as well. Aversive behaviors should be limited, as children whose parents exhibit aversive behaviors can have difficulties with emotion regulation as well as internalizing symptoms. Granting autonomy was related to reductions in depression; however, the link to reduced anxiety was not as robust. Parental withdrawal and inconsistent discipline were related to symptoms of depression. Yap et al. (2014) stated that more research is needed to determine the link between these behaviors and childhood experiences of anxiety. When working with youth with anxiety and depression, it is essential to take a thorough history and continue to observe which parental behaviors are related to child functioning and address these issues in family sessions.

A transdiagnostic approach emphasizes reviewing symptoms and their impact, rather than just considering diagnoses, which are global in nature (Ehrenreich-May & Chu, 2014). Treatment is focused and addresses key problems impeding functioning. Multicomponent programs that address common symptoms for both disorders may be advantageous for group sessions. One such program is the, EMOTION Program which is a multicomponent program, based on cognitive-behavioral techniques, to prevent and treat both anxiety and depressive symptoms in children (e.g., Martinsen et al., 2016).

EMOTION Program

Martinsen et al. (2016) developed the "EMOTION Program for Coping Kids Managing Anxiety and Depression." They recruited fifth grade children from many schools to participate in an implementation study, using the EMOTION Program Manuals for children and their parents (Kendall, Stark, Martinsen, O'Neil, & Arora, 2013; Rodriguez, Kendall, Stark, & Martinsen, 2013; Stark, Martinsen, Rodriguez, Kendall, & Arora, 2013). The program was developed for children between the ages of 8 and 12 years. Martinsen et al. selected children from over 30 schools and randomly assigned schools as the unit for receiving the intervention. The intervention uses cognitive-behavioral techniques. Parent sessions were used to deliver program material (i.e., help parents learn treatment techniques) and understand the child's perspective of anxiety and depression (Martinsen et al., 2016). The EMOTION program targets anxiety using the Coping Cat Program developed by Kendall et al. (2013) and targets depression using the Taking Action Program developed by Stark et al. (2013). Martinsen et al. (2016) combined the aforementioned programs to develop a transdiagnostic program to treat both disorders in children. Martinsen (2018) presented an overview of common mechanisms or strategies addressed by the child and parent EMOTION Programs. These included goal setting, understanding emotion-focused coping, problem-solving, cognitive restructuring, exposure and behavioral activation, and use of positive reinforcement for change. The aforementioned strategies aim to help children and parents understand emotions related to anxiety and sadness and how to regulate these emotions, detect and correct information processing errors, change child withdrawal, and improve child self-esteem. In particular, treatment targets involved helping children cope with sad and anxious feelings, reducing rumination, problem-solving for interpersonal and avoidance behavior, and exposure to reduce withdrawal associated with depression and avoidance behaviors related to fears. After participating in treatment, children reported decreased anxiety and depression, while parents reported decreases in childhood depression, but not changes in anxiety levels (Martinsen et al., 2016).

The program typically consists of 20 sessions with two individual sessions with therapists to develop individualized treatment goals for children. The sessions are typically 45–60 min per week and occur two times each week (Martinsen et al., 2016). The high number of sessions is used to enhance maintenance of treatment. Children complete homework to practice skills learned in sessions. In a series of four studies presented in her dissertation, Martinsen (2018) provided a review of the EMOTION Program, indicating it could be successfully implemented with school-age children and is feasible for use in schools. Martinsen (2018) concluded that the program was effective, but mentioned that clinicians might find the 20 sessions difficult to implement in a primary care setting. On the other hand, the treatment techniques are creative and research-based and using these in a modular approach, matching them to symptoms, may be an effective way for clinicians to use components of this program.

EMOTION Program: Key Strategies for Use with Children Martinsen et al. (2016) presented key treatment techniques for children that are included in the EMOTION Program. For instance, during an initial session, children wore dark sunglasses to see how things might look if they saw the world through dark glasses. They discussed how seeing through the glasses changed their perspective. Additionally, children learned about how the brain, body, and behavior are connected and how to use an EMOTION thermometer to see how their feelings changed based on a beach ball game they engaged in with other children and group leaders. They rated their feelings before and after the activity to see how participating in a fun game changed their mood. Children learned to be an "emotion detective" and learn how their bodily reactions were related to their thoughts and feelings and future actions. Understanding the triggers for their anxiety or depression and ways to relax helped children to understand and gain control of symptoms. Strategies the emotion detective could use included: talking to someone, reducing negative thinking (stopping negative thoughts and thinking more positively), doing something fun, and doing something that uses energy. Being an emotion detective helps children to determine where negative, self-defeating thoughts exist. The emotion detective asks if there is another way of looking at the situation or if there is evidence for a negative thought. In sum, emotion detectives are "problem-solvers" and learn to think through and find several positive solutions to anxiety provoking and stressful social situations (Martinsen, 2018; Martinsen et al., 2016).

Other cognitive strategies are used to build child skills. For example, thought bubbles are used to connect thoughts to feelings and behaviors (Martinsen et al., 2016). Children write their thoughts in the thought bubbles and learn how these thoughts are related to feelings and behaviors in different examples. Group leaders work with children to improve their self-view, and develop a positive self-schema, and begin to act in more positive ways. Children engage in "brave" actions, such as having a friend to their home. They use a "self-map" to explore their own strengths and positive capabilities (Martinsen et al., 2016). For anxiety, children make "brave plans" where they practice exposures to feared stimuli. They can do this in vivo, through writing a story of what might happen in a situation and then writing different ways to interpret the situation, so the story turns out positively with coping success. As they write their brave plan, group leaders help the child change negative self-talk to more positive self-statements. I believe components of this program may be useful for clinicians working with coaches and activity leaders in community settings, as the ideas are very easy to teach to others.

Brief Behavioral Therapy

Weersing et al. (2017) implemented behavioral techniques for children presenting with anxiety and depression called Brief Behavioral Therapy (BBT) that may be useful in primary care settings. Weersing, Gonzalez, Campo, and Lucas (2008) developed this program based on a deployment-focused approach (Weisz, 2000). This model assists in creating practice tools by moving from small pilot efficacy tests to real-world trials in service settings. Weersing et al. (2008) developed an eight-session protocol with four educational sessions, three practice sessions, and one termination and relapse prevention session. The program emphasizes problem-solving and relaxation to manage stress and anxiety and active engagement in fun life activities. Parents of younger children (ages 8–12 years) attend the sessions with the child. For older youth (13–17 years), parents attend about 50% of the sessions with their child.

Behavioral Strategies for BBT In session 1, children learn about how a small negative event can spiral into major negative feelings of anxiety and depression (Weersing et al., 2008). Parents and youth learn about the flight or fight response that is activated when an emotional spiral occurs. After this, children identify their somatic symptoms. In session 2, the clinician reviews relaxation and ideas for coping with negative mood. Three types of relaxation are presented: somatic relaxation, guided imagery, and use of pleasant and relaxing activities. Participants are taught progressive muscle relaxation and breathing, and they identify pleasant and soothing activities to improve mood. The youth is encouraged to pick one of the techniques to practice at home. In session 3, children learn problem-solving. The children make plans for coping with anxiety and depression and contract with themselves to try to employ the plans. There are workbook examples of problem-solving scenarios for youth who have difficulty with developing plans. There is homework, including mood monitoring, use of relaxation, and when appropriate, use of problem-solving strategies.

Session 4 involves setting goals that are highly enjoyable and attainable. The therapist and child review ideas for reducing avoidance of anxiety-provoking events and avoidance of social situations. Weersing et al. (2008) provided an explanation,

> Avoidance can also be a problem because we never really learn how to deal with the problems that are bothering us. You can get stuck in a serious negative spiral of feeling bad, hiding away, feeling more helpless and stressed, and then pulling back and avoiding even more. Does this make sense to you? Can you think of examples of this from your own life? This description is designed to lead into a discussion of the opposite of avoidance—graded engagement. (p. 130)

Possible goals might center on doing activities independently from parents and improving engagement with peers. Youth with anxiety might design plans that involve graded exposure (series of steps) to improve involvement in an activity. Children move from less anxiety-provoking to more anxiety-provoking tasks. Sessions 5–7 involve continual improvement on engagement plans. Youth have opportunities to practice their skills through exposure situations (e.g., anxiety, such as fear of the dark) and role play (e.g., socializing with others to lift feelings of depression). In sessions, clinicians review homework with children and problem-solve obstacles to achieving goals. The final session or eighth session involves a summary of treatment techniques, child goals, and a review of problem-solving steps in case future stressors occur. Weersing et al. (2008) provided case studies of children with comorbid anxiety and depression, to showcase the success of their program.

Real-World Trial of BBT In a randomized trial in clinical practice settings, Weersing et al. (2017) assessed outcomes for youth, ages 8 to 16 years, participating in Brief Behavioral Therapy (BBT) or Assisted Referral to Care (ARC). Children and adolescents with an array of anxiety and depressive disorders, such as separation anxiety, generalized anxiety disorder, persistent depressive disorder (dysthymia) and major depression, participated. The treatment consisted of 8–12 45-min, weekly sessions delivered by therapists (at the masters' level). Children were randomly assigned to participate in the BBT group ($n = 95$) or the ARC group ($n = 90$). Children in the BBT group participated in graded exposures to confront anxiety and stop withdrawal. They learned relaxation and problem-solving skills to relieve stress (see Weersing et al., 2008). Parents and children in the ARC group received information about symptoms, referral, and education about obtaining services. Those in the ARC group also received telephone calls to reduce barriers and encourage enrollment in services.

Results indicated that 50 of the 88 youth (about 57%) receiving BBT treatment were responders, showing reduced clinical symptoms, while 20 of the 71 youth (about 28%) who remained in the ARC group were responders (Weersing et al., 2017). There was a faster rate of improvement in symptoms for youth in the BBT compared to the ARC group. Weersing et al. (2017) concluded this was primarily due to a reduction in anxiety. The enhanced referral procedures were effective in helping youth get into mental health care (use rates of 82%), and this is important, as many parents report difficulty accessing care. Weersing et al. (2017) pointed out that cognitive restructuring was not part of treatment, and a positive impact was achieved with behavioral treatments alone. I have reviewed different treatment techniques (see Weersing et al., 2008) and feel that problem-solving and understanding emotional spirals could potentially be considered cognitive in nature. It is noteworthy that BBT treatment (Weersing et al., 2017) was delivered in settings where mental health services were co-located with medical services. This may not be common in many settings. On the other hand, Schroeder and her colleagues (e.g., Routh, Schroeder, & Koocher, 1983) have written about the positive impact of co-location and having "on-the-spot" referral and treatment for children at pediatricians' offices, and this remains a direction for consideration in the delivery of children's mental health services.

Behavioral Activation Therapy

Chu, Colognori, Weissman, and Bannon (2009) developed Behavioral Activation Therapy (BAT) for youth with anxiety and depression. Chu et al. (2009) adapted this treatment from a behavioral activation approach for adults (Jacobson, Martell, & Dimidjian, 2001). BAT involves increasing engagement in adaptive activities, decreasing engagement in activities that maintain depression, and solving problems to improve access to rewards and reduce aversive experiences (Dimidjian, Barrera, Martell, Muñoz, & Lewinsohn, 2011). Improving response-contingent positive reinforcement is at the heart of early models for remediating depressive symptoms. Improved awareness of negative self-statements and negative interpretations of events are central to this treatment. Clinicians work with clients to move in small steps toward more social activation and help the client to problem-solve to remove roadblocks to success.

Chu et al. (2009) added exposure techniques to help modify BAT for anxious youth. Although this treatment was conceptualized for young adolescents, I believe it can be modified for use with younger children. Chu et al. (2009) piloted the program with seventh and eighth graders in schools and found that the program was feasible and resulted in reduced symptoms. Chu and another group of colleagues conducted a randomized controlled trial of BAT in groups, emphasizing stopping avoidance (e.g., "anti-avoidance") and in vivo exposure to anxiety-producing events and stimuli (Chu et al., 2016). Those youth in the GBAT (Group BAT) condition showed a reduction in symptoms and impairment compared to youth assigned to a waitlist control group. Specifically, youth who participated in treatment were engaging in more pleasurable events and reported fewer negative thoughts compared to youth in the waitlist control group (Chu et al., 2016).

Increasing involvement in fun activities is a great way to engage youth in treatment. It is a relatively easy thing for many parents to begin with—as agents of change in the treatment process. Additionally, clinicians need to teach parents to recognize their child's negative thinking patterns and model more positive self-talk. Perhaps one might teach parents to recognize thinking that leads to negative emotional spirals (e.g., increasing emotions on an anxiety or sadness thermometer) characteristic of anxious and "depressogenic" cognitions. Parents can then recognize their children engaging in negative thinking and coach them to be more positive when they see these thinking processes. Learning that avoidance of feared events and stimuli are central to anxiety, while avoidance of social interactions and a lack of involvement in pleasurable activities can be central to depression may be helpful for parents. Understanding these links may help parents gain knowledge of their child's symptoms. Furthermore, understanding that small steps and successes can lead to larger ones, and that graded exposure is central to anxiety treatment is useful education for parents. Similarly, involving children in more activities, which children may resist at first, may be important to lifting feelings of depression.

The BBT program (Weersing et al., 2017), EMOTION Program (Martinsen et al., 2016), and BAT Program (Chu et al., 2009), are evidence-based tools for therapists working with children and adolescents who experience anxiety and depression. Programs that can be delivered in schools have the potential to reach many children. If techniques in successful programs are used in prevention programs, then these interventions may have the potential to either lessen symptoms or prevent or prolong the onset of symptoms (Werner-Seidler et al., 2017). The next program I discuss has been used as a universal (e.g., school-wide) prevention program for children.

Friends for Life Program

The FRIENDS for Life Program is a school-based program which aims to prevent mental health problems and boost resilience and social-emotional development in children between the ages of 7 and 12 (e. g., Iizuka, Barrett, Gillies, Cook, &

Marinovic, 2015). This program was developed by Paula Barrett who founded the Pathways Health and Research Centre in Australia. There is a group leader's and a children's workbook (Barrett, 2004a, 2004b). This program was originally developed as an anxiety prevention program and has been used as a universal prevention program to boost social and emotional skills. This program, based on cognitive-behavioral techniques, has been successful in preventing anxiety and improving coping skills and self-concept (Iizuka et al., 2015).

> The program teaches children behavioural, physiological, and cognitive strategies that enable them to identify their feelings, regulate their emotions using coping skills, identify unhelpful thoughts to replace them with more helpful thoughts, and how to face and overcome their problems and challenges with specific step plans. (Iizuka et al., 2015, p. 3)

This program has been successfully implemented in schools and is easy for teachers to administer in the classroom.

The Friends for Life Program has been evaluated in several trials with variable results (Kösters, Chinapaw, Zwaanswijk, van der Wal, & Koot, 2015). For instance, Kösters et al. (2015) evaluated the effectiveness of this program in Amsterdam with 339 children in an intervention group and 157 children in a control group. Mental health prevention workers delivered the Dutch translation of this program. Youth were between 8 and 13 years of age (mean age about 10 years, 8 months). This program was delivered during the school day and there were ten sessions, with children in the intervention group attending, on average, about nine sessions ($SD = 1.3$ sessions). Results indicated that over time children in the intervention group reported lower anxiety and depression, even at a long-term follow-up assessment (12-month follow-up). Children provided their perceptions on the *Revised Child Anxiety and Depression Scale*, which is good scale for tracking change in child report of anxiety and depression over time (Piqueras, Martín-Vivar, Sandin, San Luis, & Pineda, 2017). Child report indicated improvement in symptoms. Interestingly, teacher report did not indicate differences in anxiety and depression for the intervention group over time. Peer report did not mirror the self-report findings, indicating that more research on this program is needed (Kösters et al., 2015).

Review of School-Based Programs

Werner-Seidler et al. (2017) conducted a meta-analysis of school-based programs to prevent anxiety and depression. Werner-Seidler et al. (2017) reviewed programs for children between the ages of 5 and 19 years of age. They reviewed programs they classified as being cognitive-behavioral in nature as well as programs relying on interpersonal theory, improving well-being, and improving mindfulness. Nevertheless, a majority of the programs used CBT techniques, such as those described in this chapter. Eighty-four percent of the programs were grounded in CBT interventions. Over half of the studies these authors reviewed were universal prevention programs and under a third were indicated programs, developed for children at risk of developing anxiety and depression. School staff delivered about 35% of the programs, which is encouraging. Over half of the programs used staff who were not from the schools to deliver programming. Most of the programs were 8–12 sessions in length. Results of the meta-analysis indicated that school-based programs had positive effects after interventions had ended and at follow-up, although effect sizes were small. Unfortunately, findings indicated that 58% of the programs reviewed did not involve parents, and I think it is important to consider parent involvement in school-based programs. Some of the interventions were delivered online, and it is critical to think about the use of technology to reach youth.

Using Technology to Reach Youth

Anstiss and Davies (2015) used a text messaging program—"Reach Out, Rise Up"—with three types of weekly messages: psychoeducational, educational, and inspirational for children and adolescents between the ages of 12 and 24 years. Forty youth met screening criteria for anxiety and depression and were included in this study. Participants received the messages for 10 weeks. In weeks 5 and 10 there was not a challenge to enable youth to reflect on previous messages. Text messages were encouraging, such as, "Dont b nervous, its all bout findin ways tht wrk 4 u" (Anstiss & Davies, 2015, p. 100). A challenge example would be, "This weeks challenge is 2 try some new activities. Experiment til u find some things that make u fell gud" (Anstiss & Davies, 2015, p. 101). Participants received the same text messages beginning a week after enrolling in the program. Thus, not all participants received the same messages at the same time. Moreover, half of the youth were randomly assigned to receive a weekly telephone contact to support them with the text messaging.

Twenty-one of the 40 youth completed the Reach Out, Rise Up text messaging program (Anstiss & Davies, 2015). Participants reported decreased anxiety and depression. Furthermore, participants reported that trying new activities lifted their spirits (i.e., improved mood). Youth stated they liked to select their own activities. Becoming involved in enjoyable activities may be crucial to improving mood of youth with internalizing symptoms. All participants who completed the program thought that other children and adolescents with anxiety and depression would benefit from the program. Twelve of the 21 participants received support by telephone. Five of the 12 youth found the additional support helpful. It would have been beneficial to learn more about those who dropped out of treatment, and this study is an example of one where several dropped out, which could indicate that the treatment was highly ineffective for a subgroup of participants. Moreover, without a control or comparison group, it is not possible to conclude that the intervention and not time caused the decrease in anxiety and depression scores. For youth with cellular telephones and milder symptoms of depression and anxiety, technology such as text messaging may be a way to educate and suggest activities to improve internalizing symptoms.

Multi-Family Psychoeducational Therapy (MF-PEP)

Fristad, Ackerman, and Nick (2018) presented an adaption of Multi-Family Psychoeducational Psychotherapy (MF-PEP) for adolescents with mood disorders. MF-PEP is grounded in CBT interventions and in the notion of expressed emotion. Psychoeducation is at the heart of the program, in order to teach children and families about symptoms, ideas for treatment, and the course of a disorder. Fristad and her colleagues have used MF-PEP as an additional treatment, combined with treatment as usual, with children and their parents (Fristad, Verducci, Walters, & Young, 2009). Fristad et al. (2018) added mindfulness training, to encourage adolescents to focus on the present and observe their own emotions without judgment in the recent adaptation of their program. A feelings thermometer was used for identification of feelings and gauging their impact. Adolescents and parents learned about mood disorder symptoms, pharmacologic and other interventions, emotion regulation, problem-solving, and communication. Parents learned about mental health in relation to navigating the mental health and school systems, about negative family patterns and their relation to child symptoms and family functioning, and ways to assist their adolescent in managing his or her mood. Results indicated that participation in the program improved understanding of symptoms for both parents and adolescents and improved adaptive coping of adolescents. Fristad et al. (2018) concluded that the program could be a model for reaching and assisting teenagers and parents when teens are not in need of acute care.

As mentioned, Fristad et al. (2009) implemented MF-PEP with children between the ages of 8 and 12 years and their parents. The majority of the children in their sample had either Bipolar Disorder or depression. There were children with comorbid disorders, including anxiety, in their sample. I believe the educational model they described would be helpful for comorbid symptoms of anxiety and depression, and fits with a transdiagnostic approach (Ehrenreich-May & Chu, 2014). Children and their parents learned about symptoms, medications, tools for managing emotions, problem-solving skills, symptom management, and improving communication. Parents learned about mental health and educational systems and their role when a child has a mood disorder. Eight weekly sessions were delivered. Parent groups were facilitated by doctoral level therapists and the children received treatment from an advanced doctoral student (under supervision) and/or with a supervisor. There were clinical psychology students who participated in the children's groups. Fristad et al. (2009) concluded that the brevity of treatment enhanced completion of treatment. There was a waitlist group that received treatment as usual. The sample included a preponderance of Caucasian boys. Nonetheless, results were promising showing improved symptoms in the treatment group and improved symptoms in the waitlist group, who received the treatment after a period of 12 months. Perhaps program participation made parents better "consumers" of mental health services so that children could receive higher quality of care. Children in the waitlist group did have a nonsignificant trend toward symptom improvement, and Fristad et al. (2009) mentioned that parents who were high-functioning may be able to access psychoeducational information without participating in MF-PEP. I consider the educational component and the idea of understanding family patterns as being critical to treatment, since mood disorders run in families and are modeled by children (Garber & Weersing, 2010).

Case Study

Jason was a middle school student feeling worry about school and suffering from depression. He had completed a short stay at an inpatient treatment facility where he had learned mindfulness skills similar to those described by Fristad et al. (2018). He was working to focus on the present and understand his experience of emotions. Moreover, he was using techniques to control and reduce emotionality related to experiencing anxiety and depression. He was learning breathing techniques to slow down his reactions, then "stop and think" and gain perspective on his emotions. He was working with a mood thermometer to "dial down strong emotions" so that he could problem-solve reactions in different social situations. When he was able to not react with strong emotions, he was better able to relate to his peers and think of ways to deal with situations, such as teasing.

Jason had difficulty communicating with his parents. He was apt to withdraw from them and stay in his room. He could experience anxiety and worry in social situations, especially those involving crowds or larger groups of peers. During therapy, he was working to understand what triggered his anxiety, and how to go through it, so that he could remain in situations with peers. He worked on an anxiety hierarchy where he listed all the things about crowds that made him nervous. Then, he numbered the items in terms of how "fearful" they were for him on a scale of "0 to 100." He learned muscle relaxation and to think of his favorite vacation spot to relax. After Jason had mastered relaxation, the therapist and he went through his fear hierarchy. He needed to be relaxed in each situation. The therapist used principles developed by Rimm and Masters (1979) to develop the list of feared situations, teach relaxation, develop a hierarchy, and then go through the items in the fear hierarchy from low to high levels of anxiety while Jason was feeling relaxed. This was a successful exercise. Also, he practiced engaging in different social situations and joined an after-school club; therefore, increasing positive social behaviors was successful for Jason. His parents were educated about anxiety management and helped remind him to use his strategies (breathing, relaxation, and positive imagery) to power through anxiety-provoking social situations. His parents praised Jason's efforts and rewarded him with extra time playing computer games for successes. He showed gains in social involvement over a 2-month period.

Jason and his parents participated in family sessions to work on communicating with each other. They began to have biweekly family meetings where they went to get ice cream or a meal together and talked about family issues. Jason and his parents learned to use "I feel …" and "I think …" statements to express feelings and thoughts in a positive manner. They learned a signal phrase, "I need a moment …"

to let each other know when they needed a moment to tune into their feelings or "dial down" an emotional reaction. These techniques proved successful. Jason and his parents reported that they were talking more with each other. Jason's parents learned to help him challenge his negative thinking and try to use positive self-statements to encourage an "I can do it" state of mind.

In month two, an episode of peer teasing at school provided the impetus for a "set back" in terms of social progress for Jason. After he was teased by a male peer, Jason became sad and depressed. He retreated to his room and old coping patterns. In turn, his parents became afraid another hospitalization would occur. They stopped family meetings in order not to "rock the boat" or take a chance on worrying Jason or making him sad. Negative family patterns resumed. Further family therapy sessions, to reopen communication channels and discuss the episode at school, were needed. During these sessions, both of Jason's parents discussed their fears about him potentially requiring hospitalization. Jason was able to reassure them that he was not experiencing significant symptoms that would necessitate a hospitalization. He learned that his parents had experienced teasing and bullying at school during one of the family sessions. Next, with the therapist's assistance Jason and his parents "problem-solved" about ways to handle teasing. Ultimately, it was decided that Jason and his mother would meet with the school counselor and inform her of the teasing episodes and report the incidents to his favorite teacher. These discussions had a positive result, and the counselor met with both boys (Jason and the boy who was teasing him) to resolve issues.

In addition to working with Jason on his emotions, another approach might have been for the counselor to work with Jason and a friend to discuss how he was feeling and to strengthen his peer support, or to possibly to talk with Jason's teacher about working with children in his class to discuss the importance of friendship and not rejecting others. A different approach might be to involve Jason in more community activities so that he improved other sources of peer support, which might boost his self-confidence. Working with coaches or activity leaders to discuss Jason's anxiety and strong emotional reactions might help them understand his issues. Teaching coaches and group leaders strategies a child is working on might empower them. Then, they could assist a child, like Jason, in implementing anxiety management and other social strategies that could help Jason be more successful with peers.

Several techniques were revisited during therapy. Jason needed reminders or "booster sessions" to review mindfulness techniques for relaxing and focusing on the here and now. These were techniques he learned during a previous hospitalization. The therapist had called his previous therapist and reviewed previous interventions. Consequently, she could incorporate these interventions in his current therapy. Jason made a list of his fears for confronting peers. After this, the therapist and his parents helped talk with him and problem-solve about ways to cope with difficult social situations and his fears related to these types of situations. Jason continued to work on strategies for managing sad and anxious feelings. Jason and his therapist worked to discover negative thoughts about himself and his abilities to interact with others. Jason and his therapist found ways to counteract negative thoughts, such as by reframing the situation in a more positive light or thinking about Jason's skills and talents for coping in situations that had the potential to cause sadness or anxiety. The therapist encouraged Jason and his parents to renew their family meetings. In these meetings, they often shared upsetting feelings and discussed ways of coping with upsetting feelings providing additional support for Jason.

Conclusions

Comorbid symptoms of anxiety and depression may be common in children (Cohen et al., 2014). A transdiagnostic approach (Ehrenreich-May & Chu, 2014) relying on cognitive-behavioral and educational techniques that are successful in lessening sadness and anxiety may be helpful in treatment and improve symptoms (e.g., Fristad et al., 2009; Martinsen et al., 2016). It is important to include parents in treatment, from my point of view. Moreover, school-based prevention programs may either attenuate symptoms of anxiety and depression or perhaps even prevent their occurrence (Iizuka et al., 2015; Werner-Seidler et al., 2017). This seems to be an area for future research given the chronic and recurring course of these two disorders (Garber & Weersing, 2010; Werner-Seidler et al., 2017). Working to manage anxiety and social withdrawal using desensitization and relaxation techniques may be promising in helping a child or adolescent to "power through" difficult situations and social experiences. Moreover, helping the child to reduce the strength of anxiety- and depression-provoking emotions and reset them, in order to problem-solve different situations so that sadness and worry do not ensue, seems to be a critical skill. In the future, developing ideas about intervention components central to treatment of both disorders, which can be delivered in individual and group sessions, will be important for making positive strategies available to youth and their parents.

References

Anstiss, D., & Davies, A. (2015). 'Reach Out, Rise Up': The efficacy of text messaging in an intervention package for anxiety and depression severity in young people. *Children and Youth Services Review, 58*, 99–103. https://doi.org/10.1016/j.childyouth.2015.09.011

Barrett, P. M. (2004a). *FRIENDS for life: Group leader's manual for children*. Brisbane, Australia: Australian Academic Press.

Barrett, P. M. (2004b). *FRIENDS for Life: Workbook for children*. Brisbane, Australia: Australian Academic Press.

Chu, B. C., Colognori, D., Weissman, A. S., & Bannon, K. (2009). An initial description and pilot of group behavioral activation therapy for anxious and depressed youth. *Cognitive and Behavioral Practice, 16*(4), 408–419. https://doi.org/10.1016/j.cbpra.2009.04.003

Chu, B. C., Crocco, S. T., Esseling, P., Areizaga, M. J., Lindner, A. M., & Skriner, L. C. (2016). Transdiagnostic group behavioral activation and exposure therapy for youth anxiety and depression: Initial randomized controlled trial. *Behaviour Research and Therapy, 76*, 65–75. https://doi.org/10.1016/j.brat.2015.11.005

Chu, B. C., & Harrison, T. L. (2007). Disorder-specific effects of CBT for anxious and depressed youth: A meta-analysis of candidate mediators of change. *Child Clinical and Family Psychology Review, 10*, 352–372. https://doi.org/10.1007/s10567-007-0028-2

Cohen, J. R., Young, J. F., Gibb, B. E., Hankin, B. L., & Abela, J. R. Z. (2014). Why are anxiety and depressive symptoms comorbid in youth? A multi-wave longitudinal examination of competing etiological models. *Journal of Affective Disorders, 161*, 21–29. https://doi.org/10.1016/j.jad.2014.02.042

Cummings, C. M., Caporino, N. E., & Kendall, P. C. (2014). Comorbidity of anxiety and depression in children and adolescents: 20 years after. *Psychological Bulletin, 140*(3), 816–845. https://doi.org/10.1037/a0034733

Dimidjian, S., Barrera, M., Jr., Martell, C., Muñoz, R. F., & Lewinsohn, P. M. (2011). The origins and current status of behavioral activation treatments for depression. *Annual Review of Clinical Psychology, 7*, 1–38. https://doi.org/10.1146/annurev-clinpsy-032210-104535

Ehrenreich-May, J., & Chu, B. C. (Eds.). (2014). *Transdiagnostic mechanisms and treatment for youth psychopathology*. New York, NY: Guilford Press.

Fristad, M. A., Ackerman, J. P., & Nick, E. A. (2018). Adaptation of Multifamily Psychoeducational Psychotherapy (MF-PEP) for adolescents with mood disorders: Preliminary findings. *Evidence-Based Practice in Child and Adolescent Mental Health, 3*(4), 252–262. https://doi.org/10.1080/23794925.2018.1509031

Fristad, M. A., Verducci, J. S., Walters, K., & Young, M. E. (2009). Impact of Multifamily Psychoeducational Psychotherapy in treating children aged 8 to 12 years with mood disorders. *Archives of General Psychiatry, 66*(9), 1013–1021. https://doi.org/10.1001/archgenpsychiatry.2009.112

Garber, J., & Weersing, V. R. (2010). Comorbidity of anxiety and depression in youth: Implications for treatment and depression. *Clinical Psychology, 17*(4), 293–306. https://doi.org/10.1111/j.1468-2850.2010.01221.x

Iizuka, C. A., Barrett, P. M., Gillies, R., Cook, C. R., & Marinovic, W. (2015). Preliminary evaluation of the FRIENDS for Life Program on Students' and Teachers' Emotional States for a school in a low socio-economic status area. *Australian Journal of Teacher Education, 40*(3). Downloaded December 31, 2018, from https://doi.org/10.14221/ajte.2014v40n3.1.

Jacobson, N. S., Martell, C. R., & Dimidjian, S. (2001). Behavioral activation treatment for depression: Returning to contextual roots. *Clinical Psychology: Science and Practice, 8*(3), 255–270. https://doi.org/10.1093/clinpsy.8.3.255

Kendall, P. C., Stark, K. D., Martinsen, K., O'Neil, K. A., & Arora, P. (2013). *EMOTION: "Coping Kids" managing anxiety and depression; Group leaders manual*. Ardmore, PA: Workbook Publishing. (133 pages). ISBN: 978-1-888805-46-8.

Kertz, S. J., Sylvester, C., Tillman, R., & Luby, J. L. (2018). Latent class profiles of anxiety symptom trajectories from preschool through school age. *Journal of Clinical Child & Adolescent Psychology, 48(2)*, 316–331. https://doi.org/10.1080/15374416.2017.1295380

Kösters, M. P., Chinapaw, M. J. M., Zwaanswijk, M., van der Wal, M. F., & Koot, H. M. (2015). Indicated prevention of childhood anxiety and depression: Results from a practice-based study up to 12 months after intervention. *American Journal of Public Health, 105*(10), 2005–2013. https://doi.org/10.2105/AJPH.2015.302742

Martinsen, K. D. (2018). *Prevention of anxiety and depression in school children: The development and testing of the new transdiagnostic EMOTION intervention*. Dissertation at the University of Oslo, ISSN 1564-3991. Downloaded December 15, 2018, from http:urn.nb.no/URN;NBN:no-63798.

Martinsen, K. D., Kendall, P. C., Stark, K., & Neumer, S. P. (2016). Prevention of anxiety and depression in children: Acceptability and feasibility of the transdiagnostic EMOTION Program. *Cognitive and Behavioral Practice, 23*(1), 1–13. https://doi.org/10.1016/j.cbpra.2014.06.005

Piqueras, J. A., Martín-Vivar, M., Sandin, B., San Luis, C., & Pineda, D. (2017). The Revised Child Anxiety and Depression Scale: A systematic review and reliability generalization meta-analysis. *Journal of Affective Disorders, 218*, 17 pages. Downloaded December 15, 2018 from https://doi.org/10.1016/j/jad.2017.04.022

Rimm, D. C., & Masters, J. C. (1979). *Behavior therapy: Techniques and empirical findings* (2nd ed.). New York, NY: Academic Press.

Rodriguez, K., Kendall, P. C., Stark, K., & Martinsen, K. (2013). *Coping kids' workbook*. Ardmore, PA: Workbook Publishing. ISBN: 978-1-888805-47-5.

Routh, D. K., Schroeder, C. S., & Koocher, G. P. (1983). Psychology and primary health care for children. *American Psychologist, 38*(1), 95–98. https://doi.org/10.1037/0003-066X.38.1.95

Stark, K. D., Martinsen, K., Rodriguez, K., Kendall, P. C., & Arora, P. (2013). *Group leaders manual for parent meetings Emotion: "Coping Kids" managing anxiety and depression*. Ardmore, PA: Workbook Publishing. ISBN: 978-1-888805-50-5.

Weersing, V. R., Brent, D. A., Rozenman, M. S., Gonzalez, A., Jeffreys, M., Dickerson, J. F., … Iyengar, S. (2017). Brief behavioral therapy for pediatric anxiety and depression in primary care. *JAMA Psychiatry, 74*(6), 571–578. https://doi.org/10.1001/jamapsychiatry.2017.0429

Weersing, V. R., Gonzalez, A., Campo, J. V., & Lucas, A. N. (2008). Brief behavioral therapy for pediatric anxiety and depression: Piloting an integrated treatment approach. *Cognitive and Behavioral Practice, 15*, 126–139.

Weisz, J. R. (2000). Agenda for child and adolescent psychotherapy research: On the need to put science into practice. *Archives of General Psychiatry, 57*, 837–838. https://doi.org/10.1001/archpsyc.57.9.837

Werner-Seidler, A., Perry, Y., Calear, A. L., Newby, J. M., & Christensen, H. (2017). School-based depression and anxiety prevention programs for young people: A systematic review and meta-analysis. *Clinical Psychology Review, 51*, 30–47. https://doi.org/10.1016/j.cpr.2016.10.005

Wolk, C. B., Beidas, R. S., & Kendall, P. C. (2015). Cognitive-behavioral therapy for child anxiety confers long-term protection from suicidality. *Journal of the American Academy of Child and Adolescent Psychiatry, 54*(3), 175–179. https://doi.org/10.1016/j.jaac.2014.12.004

Yap, M. B. H., Pilkington, P. D., & Ryan, S. M. (2014). Parental factors associated with depression and anxiety in young people: A systematic review and meta-analysis. *Journal of Affective Disorders, 156*, 8–23. https://doi.org/10.1016/j.jad.2013.11.007

Chapter 4
Substance Abuse and Anxiety in Children

Introduction

Coping with a mental health and substance use problem may be a heavy burden for youth. The substance use problem may mean that many providers are not available to work with youth, necessitating inpatient treatment, which can be difficult to access. Wu et al. (2010) noted that, "… substance use disorders comorbid with anxiety disorders … tend to be more difficult to treat than substance use disorders alone" (p. 177). Erskine et al. (2015) reviewed mental health and substance use problems in youth between birth and 24 years of age. Across the globe, they found that mental health problems and substance use issues ranked sixth in terms of disease burden and quality of life lost. These problems were related to suicide attempts and suicide in youth. Substance use in those aged 10–24 years (typically beginning in adolescence and peaking around ages 20–24 years), may disrupt key changes that need to occur as youth move toward independence (Degenhardt, Stockings, Patton, Hall, & Lynskey, 2016).

The burden from alcohol and other illicit drugs is high and has become a global health concern (Degenhardt et al., 2016). Depression has figured prominently in loss of quality of life, in terms of mental health issues that co-occur with substance use (Erskine et al., 2015). Anxiety may not be as significant in its impact but is still of significant concern (Degenhardt et al., 2016). On the other hand, since depression and anxiety commonly co-occur, as do trauma and anxiety, it may be that anxiety plays a moderating role when either trauma or depression and substance use problems are present. Cicchetti and Rogosch (2018) suggested that adolescent substance use develops over time and is a result of complex interplay between biological, individual, and contextual factors, of which, psychopathology, such as anxiety, can play a role in "tipping the scales" toward substance use. Further research needs to be conducted to determine the interplay among anxiety, other mental health problems, and substance use and quality of life and morbidities for adolescents (Erskine et al., 2015).

L. Nabors, *Anxiety Management in Children with Mental and Physical Health Problems*, Springer Series on Child and Family Studies,
https://doi.org/10.1007/978-3-030-35606-4_4

Demographic factors may be linked to substance use. For example, there may be sex differences in types of anxiety disorders and substance use disorders. For example, there is some evidence that social phobia is associated with drug use for girls and cigarette smoking for boys (Wu et al., 2010). Others have reported that youth who are African American are more at risk for substance use problems (e.g., Kilpatrick et al., 2000). More research is needed to understand sex and ethnic group differences in the manifestation of anxiety disorders and comorbid substance use problems.

Risk and Resilience Factors

Many risk factors have been related to adolescent use of alcohol, cigarettes, and cannabis (Cleveland, Feinberg, Bontempo, & Greenberg, 2008). For instance, negative peer influence (e.g., use of drugs by peers) is a risk factor for substance use (Degenhardt et al., 2016). Other risk factors are witnessing violence or experiencing violence or assault (Kilpatrick et al., 2000). Choice of peer environment can influence substance use. Selecting peers that engage in substance use and risky behavior or falling into this type of peer group is associated with substance use (Jones, Epstein, Hill, Bailey, & Hawkins, 2019). The family environment of substance use can be familiar and, in turn, finding this same type of environment can occur in the teenage years (Jones et al., 2019). On the other hand, Jones et al. (2016) reported that the early teen years are optimal for prevention efforts. Starting alcohol and drug use at an early age, is a risk factor for later misuse (Degenhardt et al., 2016). Establishing positive patterns of friendships and understanding refusal skills before adolescence can mitigate risk, as association with a peer group that is using substances is strongly associated with adolescent substance use (Degenhardt et al., 2016).

Substance use disorders and anxiety tend to run in families, and have a heritability factor plus a learned behavior link (e.g., learning from a family member with substance use problems; Bountress & Chassin, 2015; Kilpatrick et al., 2000). It may be that strong family cohesion as well as family use of rewards and positive discipline are protective factors, associated with decreased chances for substance use (Cleveland et al., 2008; Jones et al., 2016). Other social protective factors are positive school involvement, laws favorable to limiting drug use and firearms, and positive peer support (Cleveland et al., 2008).

Parental Substance Use Problems

Child and adolescent internalizing problems, when a parent has a substance use problem, may be related to "… impaired parenting, family conflict, and high levels of life stress" (Bountress & Chassin, 2015, p. 275). Bountress and Chassin (2015) reported that literature on the link between internalizing problems, such as anxiety, and substance use disorders in parents has been equivocal. They did point out that children of parents with substance use disorders may be at risk for substance use disorders if they lack parental support, because internalizing problems are linked to children's relationships with their parents. Clinicians need to inquire about parental substance use problems, and make referrals for treatment as necessary. Recovery for parents could impact the family environment and thus improve child functioning (Bountress & Chassin, 2015). Assessment of family substance use is important, as it can be related to later difficulties with child involvement in environments that promote substance use (Jones et al., 2016).

Calhoun, Conner, Miller, and Messina (2015) reviewed randomized controlled trials of interventions aimed at improving functioning of parents who engaged in substance use, in order to determine what interventions were associated with improved child functioning. They reviewed 288 studies; however, only four of the studies met criteria for inclusion in their review. These studies were randomized controlled trials and had parent training incorporated in the intervention. One study provided a group of parents two sessions of training compared to standard treatment at a methadone clinic. Those parents who received "parenting training" learned behavior management skills and how to build strong relationships with their children. Parents who had the training were less likely to abuse their children and there was improved family functioning compared to performance indicators for parents who did not participate in training. Another intervention they reviewed focused on improving family communication and increasing parent knowledge of behavior management skills for positive discipline. Parents participated in sessions and children joined sessions, so parents could practice new skills with their child. At a long-term follow-up (over 10 years), male children were less likely to engage in substance use if they participated in treatment (there were not significant positive differences for females). Parents in a couples' therapy intervention, which added a parenting component, also had children with more positive outcomes. This literature review provided support for adding parent training as part of interventions to address parent substance use (Calhoun et al., 2015).

Family and Peer Influence: Developmental Cascades

Jones et al. (2016) assessed how childhood functioning was related to adult functioning in children who participated in the Seattle Social Development Project ($N = 765$ provided data for analyses). For this project, children were followed from elementary school (age 10 years) into adulthood (age 33 years). Children were interviewed at ages 10–16 and parents and teachers completed surveys. Youth completed interviews every 3 years from age 21 to age 33. Jones et al. (2016) believed that the influence of social environments impacted behavior. Consequently, how the child was functioning could "cascade" from one developmental level to another, and functioning at one level could be related to another developmental level over time.

Jones et al. (2016) defined a developmental cascade as, "… the longitudinal pathway examining how problems in individual functioning and environmental influencers spill over into other domains of functioning and into subsequent developmental periods" (p. 721).

Jones et al. (2016) proposed that personal characteristics interacted with the child's environment to influence development. Specifically, behavioral disinhibition could negatively affect a child's selection of environments (e.g., the child would select risky environments or substance using ones) and this could begin a negative cascade that could move forward into a new developmental period. Jones et al. (2016) recommended intervening in middle childhood because children could select positive peer networks and partners, whereas one enters into a family. In addition, Jones et al. (2016) found a positive family environment was protective from childhood to adulthood.

Having a family where substance use was present, then selecting peers and partners with substance use issues, was related to mental health problems in adulthood (Jones et al., 2016). Results for internalizing problems and long-term functioning were not definitive. Jones et al. (2016) did not find a relationship between internalizing problems (at ages 13 or 14 years) and negative mental health outcomes at 21 years. They did *not* find support for inter-generational transmission of anxiety, although they did report concerns for inter-generational transmission of depression. They did caution that perhaps their assessment of internalizing symptoms was not as sensitive as it could have been, as teachers provided ratings of child internalizing behaviors and parent or child ratings might have been more sensitive to these types of problems.

Anxiety Sensitivity

Another variable, related to the family environment, which can be related to later substance use, is not feeling comfortable or secure in one's family. Children who are insecure within their family may be "anxiety-sensitive." Consequently, it may be that children who grow up "unsure" in what they feel is an unstable environment, are more prone to being anxiety-sensitive and using substances to cope with anxiety. Viana and Stevens (2016) studied the link between threatening parental behaviors and substance use. They drew on literature showing that exposure to threatening and/or abusive parenting is related to substance use in adolescence (e.g., Deas, 2006). They proposed that anxiety sensitivity might moderate the relationship between threatening parenting and subsequent substance use. They anticipated that individuals who were sensitive to anxiety may have more difficulty coping with threatening behaviors and be more prone to engaging in substance use.

Viana and Stevens' (2016) participants were over 800 undergraduate students enrolled in introductory psychology courses. Their results indicated that parental threatening behavior "… was significantly positively associated with AS [anxiety sensitivity] and alcohol/tobacco illicit, and average substance use" (Viana &

Stevens, 2016, p. 216). They surmised that parental threatening behaviors may indicate that the parent is not emotionally available and may inflict pain. This lack of stability in the attachment relationship could cause feelings of worry, stress, and anxiety, which leads to high anxiety sensitivity. Teaching children who have become anxiety-sensitive to deal appropriately with physiological arousal and heightened emotions related to feelings of security may be one way to reduce their emotional insecurity and reduce risk for substance use. The link through which the anxiety works may be through trauma, and parental behaviors that are threatening may be just one example of trauma that causes anxiety.

Youth with psychopathy, who exhibit antisocial and manipulative behaviors, in addition to impulsivity, callousness, and not feeling remorse may be prone to substance use. Interestingly, those who have the aforementioned traits and anxiety sensitivity, and the emotionality that accompanies the anxiety sensitivity, may be at even higher risk for substance use (Gillen, Barry, & Bater, 2016). Teenagers with the "added" anxiety—and accompanying worry and social concerns—may engage in substance use to cope with their emotional reactivity. It may be the case that substance use allows teenagers to avoid fear or anxiety they feel. Gillen et al. (2016) found that adolescents with psychopathy and anxiety were more likely to use marijuana and alcohol. Gillen et al. (2016) recommended that researchers teach youth different problem-solving strategies as well as use motivational interviewing to help encourage youth to develop strategies to cope with their anxiety.

Impact of Traumatic Experiences

Trauma experiences are risk factors linking substance use and anxiety in children and adolescents (Cicchetti & Rogosch, 2018; Vujanovic, Farris, et al., 2018; Vujanovic, Smith, Green, Lane, & Schmitz, 2018). The link may be through the diagnosis of Post-Traumatic Stress Disorder (PTSD), which often involves considerable anxiety. Comorbid substance use and PTSD are hard to treat, and recovery can be difficult (Vujanovic, Farris, et al., 2018). Those with PTSD and substance use have higher rates of physical health problems, are more likely to be exposed to violence, have poorer social functioning, and have higher numbers of suicide attempts. Individuals with PTSD may report experiencing more significant drug cravings, while being more likely to use substances to deal with negative and unpleasant moods (Vujanovic, Farris, et al., 2018).

Anxiety sensitivity can be decreased, which, in turn, could decrease potential substance use. The anxiety that people with PTSD feel may be exacerbated by recall of traumatic experiences. Processing trauma (e.g., talking about it in a safe space with a therapist) and learning anxiety management strategies may help reduce tendencies to use substances to mask anxiety and emotional pain. Treating anxiety may diminish tendencies to relapse after substance use treatment. Cognitive Processing Therapy is often used to treat trauma, helping patients change cognitions around power, control, safety, self-esteem, trust, and intimacy (Vujanovic, Farris, et al., 2018; Vujanovic,

Smith, et al., 2018). Changing cognitions about using substances, learning to avoid cues to use substances, and processing trauma to reduce anxiety are cornerstones of treatment for individuals with PTSD and substance use problems. As mentioned, maybe using substances relieves negative affect (e.g., McHugh & Kneeland, 2019). Therefore, working on positive self-talk and thinking may help improve both anxiety symptoms and substance use.

Cognitive-behavioral techniques, such as avoiding cues (e.g., bars, parties where there is drinking) for substance use and changing thoughts about drinking, are other common interventions for treatment of substance use (Vujanovic, Smith, et al., 2018). Treatment of substance use can involve learning ways to manage cravings, learn new coping behaviors in high-risk "cue" situations, and learning to understand the links among feelings, thoughts, and substance use behaviors. Additionally, treatment can involve teaching patients to tolerate and handle stress in a new way, while reinterpreting or avoiding cues for substance use (Pagliaro & Pagliaro, 2012). Vujanovic, Smith, et al. (2018) worked with adults; nevertheless, I believe that their treatment ideas may be incorporated in treatment for adolescents.

The Complex Trauma Workgroup (CTWG) of the National Child Traumatic Stress Network identified components of interventions for trauma (Cook et al., 2005). Behavioral dysregulation or difficulty regulating emotions may be a common experience for youth who have experienced trauma, as well as for those coping with anxiety and substance use (e.g., Siegel, 2015). Other symptoms associated with trauma are difficulties with behavioral control and anxiety, dissociation (feelings of depersonalization), problems with attachments to others, poor self-concept, and difficulties with sustaining attention. Table 4.1 presents some of my ideas for treatment of complex trauma (my ideas are consistent with Cognitive Processing Therapy, Vujanovic, Farris, et al. (2018); Vujanovic, Smith, et al. (2018).

Interventions for improving affect and cognitive regulation, such as mindfulness and meditation interventions, may be especially helpful for youth who are coping with trauma, anxiety, and substance use (Siegel, 2015). Increasing self-worth and teaching youth to feel happy in interpersonal relationships may be beneficial for youth with anxiety and substance use disorders. Encouraging positive attachments with other individuals engaging in prosocial behavior and positive social activities and encouraging school involvement may help improve functioning.

School-Based Programs

Onrust, Otten, Lammers, and Smit (2016) reviewed the effectiveness of school-based programs to prevent substance use, as current research had yielded mixed or equivocal findings. Their literature review yielded 288 programs with over 400,000 participants. Programs addressed a variety of strategies to promote knowledge and build refusal and self-control skills. Among these were health education approaches, teaching refusal and social skills, using peer education to teach skills and critical information, teaching stress management, and self-esteem boosting activities.

Table 4.1 Treatment Issues and Ideas for Intervention for Trauma

Treatment issue	Ideas for intervention
Improving feelings of safety	Allow youth to express feelings and differentiate trauma experience (in the past) from current life experiences. Develop safe places at home. Use a trauma box where child can store feelings and experiences. The child can "put the lid on the box" when needed (the child can leave this with the therapist if necessary).
Improve emotion regulation and cognitive processing (e.g., attention)	Breathing, positive thinking, positive self-talk, problem-solving, meditation, mindfulness training
Integration of traumatic experiences	Allow the child or adolescent to process traumatic experiences in the therapy session. Let the child or adolescent know that what occurred is not his or her fault. Assist the child in making meaning of the experience and in grieving as the child moves on with life.
Improving relational engagement with others/ ensure positive relational experiences and attachments	Involve the child or adolescent in activities with his/her family; improve involvement in meaningful extracurricular activities; find mentors for positive attachment relationships.
Improve feelings of self-worth	Increase involvement in positive activities; help the child or adolescent develop hobbies; praise successes; take an assets-based approach to therapy.

Problem-solving and self-control strategies were emphasized by other programs. Youth in grades 8 and 9 responded well to learning refusal skills and self-control training. Those in grades 10 through 12 responded well to education emphasizing self-control as well as training in social skills (e.g., refusal skills) and problem-solving (Onrust et al., 2016). Parental involvement in programming was helpful and is recommended, as parents can monitor child behavior and continue to emphasize messages from programming at home. Onrust et al. (2016) reported that some programs were effective for different age groups. There was not a "one-size fits all" program. It may be that different programs are effective at different ages due to the different cognitive and emotional abilities for children in different age ranges.

I believe that teaching children refusal skills, along with ideas for other social activities to engage in with peers, such as going to a sports event, may improve the social acceptability of refusal. One strategy is to say "no" to using substances and not to the person(s). Another strategy is to have youth make a public commitment to not use substances. A third is to teach them about healthy alternatives to having fun with peers (e.g., cooking, going to events with peers). Research is needed to understand what works for whom. Due to the global health burden, prevention programming, in and of itself, may not be enough to limit harm to youth. As noted by Degenhardt et al. (2016), "policy levers" (p. 251) may be needed, and chief among these is making it illegal to buy or use drugs at young ages. Other legislation can restrict the availability of substances. There is a concern that low-income countries do not have the capacity to implement these policies, especially in light of the promotional efforts of alcohol and drug companies.

Social Anxiety and Substance Use in Adolescence

Earlier in this chapter, I highlighted the impact of the environment on substance use, because substance use may occur socially with others (Lemyre, Gauthier-Légaré, & Bélanger, 2019). Given this social issue, it is critical to discuss relations among shyness, social anxiety, and substance use. Lemyre et al. (2019) noted that there are similarities among shyness, social anxiety, and Social Anxiety Disorder. The underpinning similarity is self-consciousness and reticence in social situations. The aforementioned characteristics define shyness, a temperamental characteristic. This self-consciousness goes a step further with social anxiety, as the person may be worried about evaluation by others in social situations. In Social Anxiety Disorder, the fear of evaluation rises to a level that interferes with daily functioning. Social situations are tolerated with significant discomfort and/or avoided. It could be that some adolescents feel intense discomfort in social situations and "cover" their anxiety by drinking alcohol or using other types of substances. In a similar fashion, being very conscious of others may increase susceptibility to peer pressure, making a teenager who is socially anxious more apt to use substances to "fit in" with the crowd or to please a peer who is pressuring him or her to use substances.

Lemyre et al. (2019) reviewed 50 studies assessing use of tobacco, alcohol, and cannabis/other drug use. In terms of tobacco use, some studies indicated there was a negative relationship between shyness and tobacco use, while other studies did not find a relationship between these two variables. Results were similar for social anxiety and tobacco use. Some studies found a relationship, while others did not. In terms of alcohol use, findings indicated that shyness was a protective factor and was negatively related to alcohol use. Results for the relations among social anxiety and alcohol use, and Social Anxiety Disorder and alcohol use, were equivocal. Some studies showed a negative relationship, some indicated a positive relationship, and others demonstrated no relationship between the variables. Finally, in terms of cannabis and other drug use, Lemyre et al. (2019) discovered that most studies found a negative relationship between shyness and cannabis/other drug use. However, a few studies did find a positive relationship or no relationship between shyness and cannabis/other drug use. On the other hand, having a social anxiety disorder (with more severe symptoms) was positively related to cannabis and other drug use. Lemyre et al. (2019) mentioned that youth with social anxiety disorder may experience a high degree of distress in social environments and have a desire to self-medicate to cope with their distress. Clinicians need to be aware of this and work with the adolescent to find other coping mechanisms for dealing with social anxiety.

Alcohol

The most common comorbidity is alcohol use and anxiety (Birrell, Newton, Teesoson, Tonks, & Slade, 2015). Birrell et al. (2015) reported that individuals with an alcohol use disorder are "... 2.6 times more likely to have a comorbid anxiety disorder" (p. 108). Individuals with anxiety and substance use problems may be more difficult to treat (Birrell et al., 2015; Wu et al., 2010). Earlier age at first alcohol use is a risk factor for abuse as is having an anxiety disorder (Birrell et al., 2015). Birrell et al. (2015) examined a national data set in Australia and discovered that individuals with early onset agoraphobia or PTSD were more likely to have their first drink earlier that the rest of the sample. Their results indicated that the, "presence of an early onset anxiety disorder significantly increased the odds of first alcohol use in any given year by 27%" (Birrell et al. 2015, p. 111).

Arbel, Perrone, and Margolin (2018) noted that adolescents may engage in risky behaviors, like substance use, to relieve worries. Although drinking may initially decrease distress and anxiety, in the long run, as the stress-response system weakens, using the substance no longer decreases anxiety and distress. This may lead to higher levels of misuse, as efforts are made to repeat the same type of anxiety relief that used to occur in the past. Alternately, anxiety sensitivity may influence stress tolerance and substance use. It may be that youth who have higher levels of anxiety sensitivity have difficulty tolerating stressful feelings (e.g., uncomfortable mood states, distress, worry) and are likely to use alcohol to cope (Wolitzky-Taylor et al., 2015). Consequently, youth may drink to avoid feelings of distress—not knowing that chronic substance use can sensitize one's stress-response system, contributing to "heightened affective responding to stress" (McHugh & Kneeland, 2019, p. 54).

Conversely, it may be a host of factors that "tip the scales" in favor of alcohol use. In a longitudinal study in New Zealand with 1,000 adolescents (ages 16–21 years), Goodwin, Fergusson, and Horwood (2004) found a relationship between anxiety and substance use dependence. They suggested that stress relief might not solely account for the linkage of substance use and anxiety. They mentioned considering other factors that might affect the relationship, such as family factors and peer influences, which were discussed earlier in this chapter. Goodwin et al. (2004) did not believe one could point to anxiety as being causative, given the many factors that are related to substance use.

Cigarettes

Smoking has been linked to externalizing behaviors and major depression in children, and there is a modest link between smoking and anxiety disorders (Upadhyaya, Deas, Brady, & Kruesi, 2002). It is difficult to say, definitively, whether anxiety exerts an independent impact on smoking behaviors. Leventhal and Zvolenksy (2015), in a review paper in the *Psychological Bulletin*, proposed a transdiagnostic vulnerability, linking depression, anxiety, and smoking. Individuals may smoke to reduce distress and avoid states of arousal associated with anxiety or negative feelings, such as sadness, fear, and/or worry.

Fluharty, Taylor, Grabski, and Munafò (2017) reviewed the association between cigarette use, anxiety, and depression in 148 studies (the studies did not exclusively assess adolescent smoking). They found that anxiety and depression were linked to future smoking. The reverse was also true, and smoking was linked to becoming depressed and/or anxious. Even though causality was indeterminate, there was a relationship between internalizing problems and smoking (Fluharty et al., 2017). Additionally, others have found a relationship between anxiety sensitivity and adolescent smoking, suggesting that smoking can be used to cope with anxiety and its resultant physiological arousal (e.g., Bilsky, Feldner, Knapp, Rojas, & Leen-Feldner, 2016). Smoking is addictive and adolescent smoking is linked to adult smoking and significant health risks, making it important to reduce teenage smoking (Chassin, Presson, Macy, & Sherman, 2018).

Leventhal et al. (2016) assessed psychiatric comorbidity for ninth grade youth using e-cigarettes and engaging in other types of smoking. They assessed youth report of anxiety, anxiety sensitivity, depression, and mood disorders. More youth were using e-cigarettes than traditional cigarettes. For those who did use traditional cigarettes—they reported lower or "worse" mental health functioning, including internalizing problems. E-cigarette users reported mental health functioning somewhere between traditional cigarette users and nonusers (who had the most positive mental health). Youth who used both e-cigarettes and traditional cigarettes were more likely to report using alcohol and other illicit drugs.

As mentioned, family environments that are tolerant of substance use may place youth at risk (e.g., Jones et al., 2016, 2019). Parental smoking is a risk factor for child and adolescent smoking initiation (Chassin et al., 2018). It may be that parental attitudes play a role—when parents are accepting of substance use, children are more likely to initiate use. This has been found to be true for smoking initiation. Sherman, Chassin, Presson, Seo, and Macy (2009) found that mothers with more positive attitudes about smoking had children and adolescents (their sample included youth ages 10–18 years) who were more likely to initiate smoking and had more positive attitudes about smoking. These authors did not assess mental health problems, as their focus was on smoking attitudes and behaviors. More research examining relations among mental health problems and smoking is needed, as youth with mental health problems may start smoking at younger ages (Fluharty et al., 2017).

Cannabis

When one thinks about adolescent substance use, one of the foremost issues that come to mind is cannabis (marijuana) use. Rates of cannabis use have been increasing in the United States and rates have more than doubled among adolescents (Hasin et al., 2015; Peraza et al., 2019). About 20% of high school students report using cannabis and 7% of high school seniors are regular (daily or near daily) cannabis users (Hasin et al., 2015). Moreover, cannabis use has increased with trends toward legalization (Peraza et al., 2019). The main ingredient in the cannabis plant (THC, delta-9-tetrahydrocannabinol) is addictive with mood-altering (e.g., mood enhancing) effects and an impact on cognitive functioning (e.g., diminished cognitive functioning, poor academic achievement, earlier onset of psychosis; Gobbi et al., 2019).

Others have echoed the negative health impact of cannabis use (e.g., Volkow, Baker, Compton, & Weiss, 2014). Cannabis is related to smoking habits and lung problems. Cannabis use is a global health concern as well, peaking at around age 20, and after this use decreases somewhat (Degenhardt et al., 2016).

Cannabis use is related to mental health problems. Gobbi et al. (2019) examined research to understand the relationships between cannabis use at age 18 years and younger as well as the relations among cannabis use, mental health problems, and suicidality in adulthood. They discussed a link between cannabis use and major depression and experiencing suicidal ideation in adulthood. There was not a link to anxiety. They recommended improving preventive interventions that teach adolescents the risks of cannabis use as well as ways to resist and cope with peer pressure to use drugs.

Youth and adults who experience cravings, have a low distress tolerance, or perceive there are barriers to quitting cannabis use are more likely to have difficulties stopping use of this drug (Peraza et al., 2019). Barriers to quitting for young people may be loss of friends and social networks. Besides, it may be difficult for adolescents to tolerate withdrawal symptoms. Fortunately, cannabis use decreases as young people marry and enter the workforce. If cannabis use continues, young adults may fail to meet these markers of adulthood (Degenhardt et al., 2016). Cannabis use is a large problem for adolescents in our country, and is featured in the case study for this chapter.

Case Study

Tim was a 13-year-old male with social anxiety, perhaps at the level of a social anxiety disorder. He did not have friends at the small, private school he attended. He was awkward with peers and had difficulty introducing himself to other peers and interacting with them, both at school and at home in his neighborhood. Tim did not admit to having social anxiety. He did disclose that he felt "bad" that he did not "fit in" with his peers. He was a "straight 'A' student" by his and his mother's report.

Tim's brother, Jake, was originally in treatment because his grades were low and he was having fights with their father, due to missing curfew. Jake's therapy focused on working on his relationship with his father and following curfews and limits at home. Jake was always very reticent to talk during therapy sessions. He was often angry and said he did not want to participate. He was able to admit that his older friends were taking him to "parties" and this might be related to his falling grades. He did concede that he was upset about altercations with his father. Jake prematurely ended therapy and never fully engaged in treatment.

About 6 months after Jake had stopped coming to treatment, Tim's mother brought him for a session. His mother was very upset because Tim had been caught using marijuana at school. He was suspended. The therapist referred Tim for an evaluation with his pediatrician or health professionals specializing in substance use for teenagers. Unfortunately, his mother did not follow through with this. Tim was reticent about talking. He was defensive and said he smoked pot with his friends one time and now he was cool. Tim said that he had gained a friendship group. Tim felt that using marijuana helped relieve his worries and was a way to gain acceptance from his friends (Arbel et al., 2018). Tim missed future sessions.

His mother came to a session and said she found marijuana pipes in his room. She said Tim admitted he smoked and drank daily. The therapist referred Tim for emergency evaluation, for substance dependence. His mother was now very alarmed and took him to a treatment center. Tim was admitted and remained at the center for 2 months.

After being released from treatment, this therapist referred Tim to a substance abuse counselor and group therapy for substance abuse. Sessions were four times a week. After 2 weeks, Tim began missing sessions. He did not attend group therapy or Alcoholics Anonymous (AA) meetings. He used to attend AA meetings with other group members from his treatment center. He missed school—he was now enrolled in a public school. He still "hung out" with his friends. He was dealing and smoking marijuana or as he said, "pot." It was discovered in his backpack and he was expelled from the public school. His mother called their therapist and said Tim mentioned he needed the drugs and liquor to feel less anxious and relate to his friends. He used the liquor and marijuana to be "chill" and "cool." It helped him feel like he was doing something that was popular. Although the therapist and groups at the treatment center had provided education and information about the risks of substance use and the importance of disengaging with dealers and risky peer groups, Tim felt he could not follow this guidance.

His mother was very upset for her child. Tim was referred for evaluation and treatment for his substance abuse problem. Referrals for three other therapists who could work with Tim on substance use issues, improving social skills, and coping with his anxiety around his peers were provided. His mother considered evaluation at a nearby hospital that specialized in mental health issues for teens. This case was referred several times, due to Tim's ongoing substance use and inability to maintain his sobriety. His pediatrician recommended referral as well, because he believed Tim needed specialists to treat his comorbid mental health issues. Some issues that could be addressed through therapy, included social skills deficits related to his anxiety and Tim would need to learn to engage in social interactions and remove himself from peers engaging in delinquent behavior (Swan & Kendall, 2016). Working with Tim to improve academic performance, which had fallen, would help as well. Correspondingly, it would be important to assess family functioning, as this factor can be related to social anxiety in youth (Swan & Kendall, 2016).

I believe that Multisystemic Family Therapy (MST) may be a good modality for treating youth with substance use and anxiety problems because individualized treatment and comprehensive services to address school and family problems are provided in the individual's natural environment (Henggeler et al., 1999). The reader is referred to Henggeler's body of work, including the book, *Multisystemic Therapy for Antisocial Behavior in Children and Adolescents: Second Edition* (Henggeler, Schoenwald, Borduin, Rowland, & Cunningham, 2009) to learn more about interventions associated with this treatment approach. The case management and therapy "when needed in real life" approach that is associated with MST may have made this a good treatment avenue for Tim. Perhaps Tim might benefit from home-based MST after his sobriety was assured (e.g., Henggeler et al., 1999). The MST approach would allow for treatment in multiple environments that impact Tim (Swan & Kendall, 2016). Tim might benefit from participating in a group for youth with substance use problems or perhaps participating in a day treatment program.

Tim had a history of difficulty regulating his emotions, often due to his anxiety and lack of self-calming skills. These are common variables associated with internalizing problems and substance use disorders (Sloan et al., 2017). As part of treatment, Tim may need to learn to better regulate his emotions and to learn to feel calm and decrease his anxiety, without turning to substance use. This may be an essential component of treatment, as emotion regulation has been a factor related to adolescent substance use (e.g., Siegel, 2015). Mindfulness and meditation training may improve emotion regulation and may help teenagers learn calming skills and to remain "present-centered." If it is determined that family members lack these skills, then expanding treatment to them may be beneficial in teaching them to regulate their emotions and self-soothe (Siegel, 2015).

The medications that are used to treat anxiety, such as Sertraline and Buspar, may not be possible to use when a patient has substance use problems. Moreover, although treatment of anxiety is often on an outpatient basis, treatment of substance use may need to occur in an inpatient setting. It may be that therapists in the hospital could review anxiety management techniques, such as exposure, cognitive restructuring (changing negative thoughts to more "can do" thoughts), and using positive self-talk and positive imagery. Managing cues for anxiety and cues for drinking may be different. Whereas one goes through or powers through anxiety, the reverse may be true for cues to use substances, which should be avoided. Teaching a child to differentiate these cues is important. When social anxiety underlies substance use, teaching the child social skills and how to navigate social situations becomes valuable. At the same time, teaching the adolescent to avoid those friends and situations that lead to substance use is an equally critical component of treatment.

Resources for Clinicians

Pagliaro and Pagliaro (2012, 2020) suggested using interventions specific to the client's presenting problems and treatment needs. For substance abuse, intervention to begin sobriety is a first step. Cognitive therapy may be needed to help the adolescent replace irrational thoughts with positive, realistic, and self-enhancing thoughts. Continued counseling and therapy to deal with feelings and past experiences, or trauma (if present), may be indicated. Behavioral therapy, including contingency management, to avoid negative stimuli that serve as cues to abuse substances may be helpful. Therapists should consider family therapy and individual treatment, while having an empathic approach centering on the youth's needs and presenting problems. Pagliaro and Pagliaro (2012) recommended checking for and addressing trauma in therapy. They recommended building self-esteem, empowering youth, and encouraging youth participation in peer and self-help groups. Ensuring that after-care with specialists in substance use is arranged, to prevent relapse, is critical. Many referral attempts may be needed, especially if a parent is resistant to referrals, as was the case for Tim's mother (see our case study). In their books, Pagliaro and Pagliaro (2012, 2020) detail different treatment and prevention programs that will improve knowledge of clinicians interested in treatment of substance use disorders. Another recent reference, detailing treatment, is the book entitled, "*Treating Adolescent Substance Use: A Clinician's Guide*," which was edited by Welsh and Hadland (2019).

Conclusions

This chapter reviews information about substance use and anxiety in youth, with a focus on three areas: alcohol, cigarette, and cannabis use. There are a host of other substances that teenagers (and some children) misuse, and the reader is directed toward the Substance Abuse and Mental Health Services Administration's evidence-based practice center website (see https://www.samhsa.gov/ebp-resource-center) to learn more about successful, evidence-based treatments for substance use for youth in different age ranges. It is noteworthy that more research on anxiety and substance use disorders in adolescents is needed. Prevention programs, delivered in the early middle school years, may be an avenue for teaching refusal and social skills before problems begin. Targeting children with social anxiety for substance use prevention messages may be crucial, as they may drink to cover anxiety. Likewise, understanding the link between substance using environments (family and peer) and substance use is critical and remains an area for research and intervention.

References

Arbel, R., Perrone, L., & Margolin, G. (2018). Adolescents' daily worries and risky behaviors: Buffering role of support seeking. *Journal of Clinical Child & Adolescent Psychology, 47*(6), 900–911. https://doi.org/10.1080/15374416.2016.1169536

Bilsky, S. A., Feldner, M. T., Knapp, A. A., Rojas, S. M., & Leen-Feldner, E. W. (2016). The roles of sex, anxious reactivity to bodily arousal, and anxiety sensitivity in coping motives for cigarette smoking among adolescents. *Experimental and Clinical Psychopharmacology, 24*(3), 147–155. https://doi.org/10.1037/pha0000071

Birrell, L., Newton, N. C., Teesson, M., Tonks, Z., & Slade, T. (2015). Anxiety disorders and first alcohol use in the general population. Findings from a nationally representative sample. *Journal of Anxiety Disorders, 31*, 108–113. https://doi.org/10.1016/j.janxdis.2015.02.008

Bountress, K., & Chassin, L. (2015). Risk for behavior problems in children of parents with substance abuse problems. *American Journal of Orthopsychiatry, 85*(3), 275–286. https://doi.org/10.1037/ort0000063

Calhoun, S., Conner, E., Miller, M., & Messina, N. (2015). Improving the outcomes of children affected by parental substance abuse: A review of randomized controlled trials. *Substance Abuse and Rehabilitation, 6*, 15–24. https://doi.org/10.2147/SAR.S46439

Chassin, L., Presson, C. C., Macy, J. T., & Sherman, S. J. (2018). Cigarette smoking from adolescence to adulthood: Findings from the Indiana University Smoking Survey. In H. E. Fitzgerald & L. I. Puttler (Eds.), *Alcohol use disorders: A developmental science approach to etiology* (pp. 237–249). New York, NY: Oxford University Press.

Cicchetti, D., & Rogosch, F. A. (2018). A developmental psychopathology perspective on substance use: Illustrations from the research on child maltreatment. In E. Fitzgerald & L. I. Puttler (Eds.), *Alcohol use disorders: A developmental science approach to etiology* (pp. 17–29). New York, NY: Oxford University Press.

Cleveland, M. J., Feinberg, M. E., Bontempo, D. E., & Greenberg, M. T. (2008). The role of risk and protective factors in substance use across adolescence. *Journal of Adolescent Health, 43*(2), 157–164. https://doi.org/10.1016/j/jadolhealth.2008.01.015

Cook, A., Spinazzola, J., Ford, J., Lanktree, C., Blaustein, M., Cloitre, M., … van der Kolk, B. (2005). Complex trauma in children and adolescents. *Psychiatric Annals, 35*(5), 390–398. https://doi.org/10.3928/00485713-20050501-05

Deas, D. (2006). Adolescent substance abuse and psychiatric comorbidities. *Journal of Clinical Psychiatry, 67*, 18–23.

Degenhardt, L., Stockings, E., Patton, G., Hall, W. D., & Lynskey, M. (2016). Substance use in young people 1: The increasing global health priority of substance use in young people. *Lancet Psychiatry, 3*, 251–264. https://doi.org/10.1016/S2215-0366(15)00508-8

Erskine, H. E., Moffitt, T. E., Copeland, W. E., Costello, E. J., Ferrari, A. J., Patton, G., … Scott, J. G. (2015). A heavy burden on young minds: The global burden of mental and substance use disorders in children and youth. *Psychological Medicine, 45*(7), 1551–1563. https://doi.org/10.1017/S0033291714002888

Fluharty, M., Taylor, A. E., Grabski, M., & Munafò, M. R. (2017). The association of cigarette smoking with depression and anxiety: A systematic review. *Nicotine and Tobacco Research, 19*(1), 3–13. https://doi.org/10.1093/ntr/ntw140

Gillen, C. T. A., Barry, C. T., & Bater, L. R. (2016). Anxiety symptoms and coping motives: Examining a potential path to substance use-related problems in adolescents with psychopathic traits. *Substance Use and Misuse, 51*(14), 1920–1929. https://doi.org/10.1080/10826084.2016.1201510

Gobbi, G., Atkin, T., Zytynski, T., Wang, S., Askari, S., Boruff, J., … Mayo, N. (2019). Association of cannabis use in adolescence and risk of depression, anxiety, and suicidality in young adulthood a systematic review and meta-analysis. *JAMA Psychiatry, 76*(4), 426–434. https://doi.org/10.1001/jamapsychiatry.2018.4500

Goodwin, R. D., Fergusson, D. M., & Horwood, L. J. (2004). Association between anxiety disorders and substance use disorders among young persons: Results of a 21-year longitudinal study. *Journal of Psychiatric Research, 38*, 295–304. https://doi.org/10.1016/j.psychires.2003.09.002

Hasin, D. S., Saha, T. D., Kerridge, B. T., Goldstein, R. B., Chou, S. P., Zhang, H., … Grant, B. F. (2015). Prevalence of marijuana use disorders in the United States between 2001-2002 and 2012-2013. *JAMA Psychiatry, 75*(12), 1235–1242. https://doi.org/10.1001/jamapsychiatry.2015.1858

Henggeler, S. W., Rowland, M. D., Randall, J., Ward, D. M., Pickrel, S. G., Cunningham, P. B., … Santos, A. B. (1999). Home-based multisystemic therapy as an alternative to hospitalization of youths in psychiatric crisis: Clinical outcomes. *Journal of the American Academy of Child & Adolescent Psychiatry, 38*(11), 1331–1339. https://doi.org/10.1097/00004583-199911000-00006

Henggeler, S. W., Schoenwald, S. K., Borduin, C. M., Rowland, M. D., & Cunningham, P. B. (2009). *Multisystemic therapy for antisocial behavior in children and adolescents* (2nd ed.). New York, NY: Guilford Press.

Jones, T. M., Epstein, M., Hill, K. G., Bailey, J. A., & Hawkins, J. D. (2019). General and specific predictors of comorbid substance use and internalizing problems from adolescence to age 33. *Prevention Science, 20*(5), 705–714. https://doi.org/10.1007/s11121-018-0959-5

Jones, T. M., Hill, K. G., Epstein, M., Lee, J. O., Hawkins, D., & Catalans, R. F. (2016). Understanding the interplay of individual and social-developmental factors in the progression of substance use and mental health from childhood to adulthood. *Development and Psychopathology, 28*(3), 721–741. https://doi.org/10.1017/S0954579416000274

Kilpatrick, D. G., Acierno, R., Saunders, B., Resnick, H. S., Best, C. L., & Schnurr, P. P. (2000). Risk factors for adolescent substance abuse and dependence data from a national sample. *Journal of Consulting and Clinical Psychology, 68*(1), 19–30.

Lemyre, A., Gauthier-Légaré, A., & Bélanger, R. E. (2019). Shyness, social anxiety, social anxiety disorder, and substance use among normative adolescent populations: A systematic review. *American Journal of Drug and Alcohol Abuse, 45*(3), 230–247. https://doi.org/10.1080/00952990.2018.1536882

Leventhal, A. M., Strong, D. R., Sussman, S., Kirkpatrick, M. G., Unger, J. B., Barrington-Trimis, J. L., & Audrain-McGovern, J. (2016). Psychiatric comorbidity in adolescent electronic and conventional cigarette use. *Journal of Psychiatric Research, 73*, 71–78. https://doi.org/10.1016/j.jpsychires.2015.11008

Leventhal, A. M., & Zvolensky, M. J. (2015). Anxiety, depression, and cigarette smoking: A transdiagnostic vulnerability framework to understanding emotion–smoking comorbidity. *Psychological Bulletin, 141*(1), 176–212. https://doi.org/10.1037/bu10000003

McHugh, R. K., & Kneeland, E. T. (2019). Affective vulnerability in substance use disorders. *Current Opinion in Psychiatry, 30*, 54–58. https://doi.org/10.1016/j.copsyc.2019.01.011

Onrust, S. A., Otten, R., Lammers, J., & Smit, F. (2016). School-based programmers to reduce and prevent substance use in different age groups: What works for whom? Systematic review and meta-regression analysis. *Clinical Psychology Review, 44*, 45–59. https://doi.org/10.1016/j.cpr.2015.11.002

Pagliaro, L. A., & Pagliaro, A. M. (2012). *Handbook of child and adolescent drug and substance abuse: Pharmacological, developmental, and clinical considerations*. Hoboken, NJ: Wiley and Sons. ISBN: 978-0-0470-63906-1.

Pagliaro, L. A., & Pagliaro, A. M. (2020). *Child and adolescent drug and substance abuse: A comprehensive reference guide. First Ed.* New York, NY: Routledge. ISBN: 978-1-138-54215-0.

Peraza, N., Smit, T., Garey, L., Manning, K., Buckner, J. D., & Zvolensky, M. J. (2019). Distress tolerance and cessation-related cannabis processes: The role of cannabis use coping motives. *Addictive Behaviors, 90*, 164–170. https://doi.org/10.1016/j.addbeh.2018.10.047

Sherman, S. J., Chassin, L., Presson, C., Seo, D.-C., & Macy, J. T. (2009). The intergenerational transmission of implicit and explicit attitudes toward smoking: Predicting adolescent smoking initiation. *Journal of Experimental Social Psychology, 45*(2), 313–319. https://doi.org/10.1016/j.jesp.2008.09.012

Siegel, J. P. (2015). Emotional regulation in adolescent substance use disorders: Rethinking risk. *Journal of Child and Adolescent Substance Abuse, 24*(2), 67–79. https://doi.org/10.1080/1067828X.2012.761169

Sloan, E., Hall, K., Moulding, R., Bryce, S., Mildred, H., & Staiger, P. K. (2017). Emotion regulation as a transdiagnostic treatment construct across anxiety, depression, substance, eating and borderline personality disorders: A systematic review. *Clinical Psychology Review, 57*, 141–163. https://doi.org/10.1016/j.cpr.2017.09.002

Swan, A. J., & Kendall, P. C. (2016). Fear and missing out: Youth anxiety and functional outcomes. *Clinical Psychology: Science and Practice, 23*, 417–435. https://doi.org/10.1111/cpsp.12169

Upadhyaya, H. P., Deas, D., Brady, K. T., & Kruesi, M. (2002). Cigarette smoking and psychiatric comorbidity in children and adolescents. *Journal of the American Academy of Child & Adolescent Psychiatry, 41*(11), 1294–1305. https://doi.org/10.1097/00004583-200211000-00010

Viana, A. G., & Stevens, E. N. (2016). Parental threatening behaviors and offspring substance use: The moderating role of anxiety sensitivity. *Journal of Child and Adolescent Substance Abuse., 25*(3), 212–221. https://doi.org/10.1080/1067828X.2014.926848

Volkow, N. D., Baker, R. D., Compton, W. M., & Weiss, S. R. (2014). Adverse health effects of marijuana use. *New England Journal of Medicine, 370*, 2219–2227. https://doi.org/10.1056/NEJMra1402309

Vujanovic, A. A., Farris, S. G., Bartlett, B. A., Lyons, R. C., Haller, M., Colvonen, P. J., & Norman, S. B. (2018). Anxiety sensitivity in the association between posttraumatic stress and substance use disorders: A systematic review. *Clinical Psychology Review, 62*, 37–55. https://doi.org/10.1016/j.cpr.2018.05.003

Vujanovic, A. A., Smith, L. J., Green, C. E., Lane, S. D., & Schmitz, J. M. (2018). Development of a novel, integrated cognitive-behavioral therapy for co-occurring posttraumatic stress and substance use disorders: A pilot randomized clinical trial. *Contemporary Clinical Trials, 65*, 123–129. https://doi.org/10.1016/j.cct.201712.013

Welsh, J. W., & Hadland, S. E. (Eds.). (2019). *Treating adolescent substance use: A clinician's guide*. Basel: Springer Nature. https://doi.org/10.1007/978-3-030-01893-1

Wolitzky-Taylor, K., Guillot, C. R., Pang, R. D., Kirkpatrick, M. G., Zvolensky, M. J., Buckner, J. D., & Leventhal, A. M. (2015). Examination of anxiety sensitivity and distress tolerance as transdiagnostic mechanisms linking multiple anxiety pathologies to alcohol use problems in adolescents. *Alcoholism, Clinical and Experimental Research, 39*(3), 532–539. https://doi.org/10.1111/acer.12638

Wu, P., Goodwin, R. D., Fuller, C., Liu, X., Comer, J. S., Cohen, P., & Hoven, C. W. (2010). The relationship between anxiety disorders and substance use among adolescents in the community: Specificity and gender differences. *Journal of Youth and Adolescence, 39*(2), 177–188. https://doi.org/10.1007/s10964-008-9385-5

Chapter 5
Autism Spectrum Disorder and Anxiety in Children

Introduction

Anxiety can be very debilitating for children with Autism Spectrum Disorders (ASD), and children and adolescents with ASD may have increased risk of anxiety disorders (van Steensel, Bögels, & Perrin, 2011; van Steensel & Heeman, 2017). ASD is characterized by different levels of impairment in communication, social interaction, and having stereotyped behaviors and interests (White et al., 2015). ASD is a lifelong disability with persistent deficits in social skills, communication deficits, and stereotypies—restricted, repetitive interests, and behaviors (American Psychiatric Association or DSM-V, 2013; Cunningham & Schreibman, 2008). One percent of children have ASD (DSM-V, 2013); however, rates vary across studies (Volkmar et al., 2014). The variation may be due to the broad array of symptoms exhibited by children with ASD. Rates of autism are thought to be increasing, perhaps because professionals are better able to identify the symptoms of this disorder (Kulage, Smaldone, & Cohn, 2014).

Approximately 40% of youth with ASD may present with an anxiety disorder (van Steensel et al., 2011; van Steensel & Heeman, 2017). Prevalence rates show a broad range across studies (from approximately "11–84%,", Ozsivadjian, Knott, & Magiati, 2012, p. 108). In fact, van Steensel and Heeman (2017) reported that children with ASD had higher levels of anxiety than children with externalizing problems, and that anxiety could increase with age. The anxiety symptoms children with ASD experience may compound social and communication deficits as well as increase stereotypies (White et al., 2015). There is some debate about whether anxiety is a feature of ASD or anxiety disorders co-occur with ASD (White et al., 2015). Kerns and Kendall (2012) proposed that ASD and anxiety disorders are different conditions, and this is the position from which this chapter was developed. It is imperative to remember that children with comorbid mental health problems may

L. Nabors, *Anxiety Management in Children with Mental and Physical Health Problems*, Springer Series on Child and Family Studies,
https://doi.org/10.1007/978-3-030-35606-4_5

present different symptoms and respond differently to treatment (e.g., Caron & Rutter, 1991), and thus understanding the evidence base and how to apply it in different scenarios may be a hallmark of good clinical practice.

Typical and Atypical Presentation of Symptoms in Children with ASD

Kerns and Kendall (2012) mentioned that research on anxiety and ASD has produced inconsistent or mixed results. This may be due to variability in samples (there are many conditions under the ASD umbrella as well as the anxiety umbrella) and due to differences in methodologies across studies. Nonetheless, they concluded that anxiety does coexist with ASD and may have typical versus atypical presentations. In a more recent study, White et al. (2015) used an anxiety survey and compared child (ages 7–17 years, mean age of about 11 years) and parent reports of anxiety for a sample of children with only anxiety and a sample of children with ASD and anxiety. Their results were inconclusive, as the data did not fit the structure of the surveys they used with the groups. However, I believe that results weremay have been inconclusive because of the many presentations of ASD and the many types of anxiety symptoms that children can face.

Anxiety may be manifested in increased behavioral reactivity and stereotypies in youth with ASD. Understanding each individual and his or her symptoms becomes central to designing behavioral interventions to help youth. In discussing results of a meta-analysis, van Steensel and Heeman (2017) supported the idea that anxiety faced by children with ASD may have a typical presentation and an atypical one, likely related to sensory preferences and reactions ("sensitivities") and social difficulties, providing further support for Kerns and Kendall's (2012) ideas about typical and atypical symptoms.

Because the presentation of symptoms may not "match" traditional assessment tools (White et al., 2015) qualitative methods may provide critical data on anxiety in youth with ASD. Ozsivadjian et al. (2012) conducted focus groups with parents to determine triggers of anxiety and sources of anxiety for youth with ASD. Their results indicated the following seven potential triggers:

1. changes or disruptions in routines,
2. social triggers (e.g., fear of being ridiculed, being a focus of others' attention),
3. specific fears/phobias that were typical (e.g., injections, spiders),
4. atypical fears (e.g., "… chocolate coming out of his belly button after watching the film *Charlie and the Chocolate Factory*", Ozsivadjian et al., 2012, p. 112),
5. sensory triggers (e.g., loud noises, too many voices, smells),
6. being prevented from carrying out stereotypies or engaging in preferences, and
7. too many social demands or expectations.

When faced with these triggers, children could experience anxiety, which was then manifested in negative (challenging) behaviors, engaging in sensory behavior (e.g., nail-biting, hand-biting), performing repetitive behaviors, attempts to avoid a stimulus, and physiological symptoms (e.g., "white, clammy, black eyes", Ozsivadjian et al., 2012, p. 113). Parents mentioned that their children often did not have the verbal skills to discuss triggers. By the time parents saw anxious behaviors it was difficult to reduce symptoms (as symptoms were high and debilitating). Some of the parents also mentioned that their children reported negative cognitions or engaged in negative self-talk, such as "… people don't like me, I am totally useless" (Ozsivadjian et al., 2012, p. 114). Atypical presentations of anxiety often were triggered by changes in routine or social situations that children who were developing typically might find pleasing, such as a holiday celebration. Parents reported feeling guilty because they could not help their child reduce his or her anxiety. Ozsivadjian et al. (2012) did conduct a small group with four boys and found that the boys' comments were consistent with information provided by their parents.

Kerns et al. (2014) assessed anxiety symptoms in youth with ASD for 59 youth (ages 7–17, mean age of about 10 years) with mild delays in cognitive functioning (IQ greater than 60). Youth with ASD presented with typical (17%) and atypical anxiety (15%), and sometimes both types of anxiety (31%). Atypical fears included fears of loud sounds and unusual phobias (fear of mechanical objects). Kerns et al. (2014) mentioned that these fears or phobias could be tied to atypical sensory experiences. Children with ASD also may have fears of social situations and rejection. Worries may also occur around changes in routine or the daily environment. These worries or fears could be related to perseverative and obsessive behaviors (restricted and unique patterns of interests). Children with ASD may be driven by rule-governed behaviors (e.g., compulsive or ritualistic behaviors), such as eating only one color of food. They can experience distress when any changes to rule-governed behaviors occur. Other researchers have reported that anxiety may be linked to an insistence on sameness for children with ASD (Gotham et al., 2013; Vasa & Masurek, 2015). Kerns et al. (2014) mentioned that negative thoughts have been related to anxiety in children. Interventions should target negative thoughts, if the therapist finds this style of thinking is linked to anxiety. A point of interest is that Kerns et al. (2014) stated that may anxiety symptoms may not meet DSM (2013) criteria for an anxiety disorder; yet, these symptoms should be targets of treatment.

Interventions

Impact of Cognitive Behavioral Therapy (CBT) Interventions Sukhodolsky, Bloch, Panza, and Reichow (2013) conducted a meta-analysis to review evidence from studies using CBT to treat anxiety in children and adolescents with ASD. They assessed treatment research where there were comparison/control conditions. Most participants had IQs in the range of 70 or higher. We lack information about effective ways to help children with ASD and with lower cognitive abilities cope with anxiety. Sukhodolsky et al. (2013) extracted eight studies for review. In these studies, a variety of anxiety management interventions were used, either during individual or group sessions. The majority of programs (n = 6) presented interventions that helped children overcome anxiety using exposure. Children learned calming strategies to help them reduce their anxiety symptoms before they went through fear associated with anxiety-provoking events or stimuli. Parent and clinician ratings from these studies indicated decreased anxiety for children and adolescents.

Sukhodolsky et al. (2013) did note that it might be difficult for parents to differentiate ASD symptoms from anxiety, especially if symptoms revolved around a need for sameness or exhibiting repetitive behaviors. Wood, Drahota, Sze, Har, et al. (2009) and Sukhodolsky et al. (2013) reported that child report of symptoms might not indicate as much positive change compared to adult reports. It may be that the CBT improves avoidance, which parents interpret as anxiety reduction. Children may still feel anxious and consequently they may not have the same interpretation. This remains an area for future investigation. Sukhodolsky et al. (2013) recommended that future studies examine treatment versus attention only conditions, and this seems to be a fruitful area for research. They speculated that anxiety and social skills deficits were interrelated and treatment of these interrelated issues could improve functioning, noting that three of the studies in their review had social skills training as part of the intervention.

Visual Schedules and Scripts Fear of change in routine(s) and fear of socializing are two fears that may cause symptoms of anxiety in children and adolescents with ASD. Interventions to make changes in routine more evident to youth, through use of visual schedules may reduce anxiety related to changes in routines or schedules. I think visual schedules with reinforcement for anxiety coping (e.g., reinforcement of calm behaviors) and following a new schedule may be helpful interventions. Using visual schedules to depict change would be an intervention that uses an asset-based approach, because youth with ASD may have relatively stronger visual skills (Mesibov & Shea, 2010). A visual schedule typically depicts an upcoming sequence of events using images, pictures, or photographs (Knight, Sartini, & Spriggs, 2015; Mesibov, Browder, & Kirkland, 2002; Mesibov & Shea, 2010). Visual schedules can depict social scripts that can make anxiety-provoking social situations more manageable for children with ASD. The scripts can provide ideas for behaviors in different social situations (Cho, Noor, & Sonoyama, 2017). They may detail steps for managing anxiety as well. Knight et al. (2015) mentioned that visual schedules work well for individuals with ASD who have differing skill levels, age levels (preschool through high school), for a variety of behaviors, with a variety of reinforcers, and have been implemented in self-contained classrooms, general classrooms, and other community settings. Visual schedules may be ineffective, however, unless combined with reinforcement for completing the activities depicted in the schedule (Waters, Lerman, & Hovanetz, 2009).

In order to understand triggers for anxiety and resulting stereotypic behaviors, it can be beneficial to conduct a functional analysis of behavior (see Gresham, Watson, & Skinner, 2001 for information on conducting a functional behavioral assessment). A functional analysis of behavior involves understanding the antecedents of a behavior (e.g., triggers), the behavior itself, and the consequences that serve to maintain a behavior. For instance, I have worked with cases where youth with ASD exhibit self-injurious stereotypies, such as hand-biting, when social demands are placed on them. In these situations, careful interviews with adults in educational and residential settings were needed to understand the "triggers" or precursors to stereotypic behaviors that might cause self-harm. If social demands are discovered as triggers, therapists may opt to develop visual scripts, with stories and illustrations to describe what to do and how to cope with environmental changes. Scripts may reduce anxiety by providing ideas about how to engage in stressful social situations. This allows children to understand what to do, and they may experience reduced worry. The visual nature of scripts also allows children with ASD to work from their visual strengths in learning new skills.

Sensory Oversensitivity Youth with ASD may experience sensory over-sensitivity and sensory avoidance (Vasa & Masurek, 2015). For example, some youth may be oversensitive to sounds. They may benefit from sensory integration training, as well as receiving reinforcement if they do not avoid sounds that make them uncomfortable. Lane, Reynolds, and Dumenci (2012) found that children with ASD may recover more slowly from challenging sensory experiences compared to children who are developing typically and that they may experience anxiety related to sensory sensitivity. Hypersensitivity and the need for sameness may be related in children with ASD. Interestingly, Black et al. (2017) found hypersensitivity was related to specific phobia and separation anxiety for youth with ASD. Exposure with rewards can be advantageous in combatting anxiety related to sensory experiences. Helping children, who are sensitive and likely to experience sensory overload, predict that there will be anxiety during the day and predicting that they can cope with the anxious feelings and gain rewards, such as time to engage in preferred activities, may encourage children to work through their anxiety. Teaching self-calming techniques, such as breathing and relaxation (e.g., muscle relaxation), may help children to "reset" physiologically, reducing arousal so that they can focus on coping with novel or anxiety-producing experiences.

Intervention Program: Secret Agent Society Sauvé, O'Haire, Hall, Lane, and Hudson (2018) implemented the Secret Agent Society (SAS), which was developed by Beaumont (e.g., Beaumont & Sofronoff, 2008). Twenty-four families participated in the intervention (six children in four groups). Children were between 8 and 13 years. This intervention had both child and parent groups. Children learned how to cope with bullying, play with others, have conversations, and use appropriate nonverbal behaviors (e.g., posture, eye contact). In addition, children learned anger/emotion management and anxiety management strategies. Parents learned these techniques as well. Children played a computer game, which allowed them to practice skills learned in their groups at home. Children could select emotional self-regulation strategies from a list of ideas. Children could earn weekly prizes if they completed their practice assignments at home.

Sauvé et al. (2018) held sessions over 9 weeks, and there were "practice missions" or homework between sessions where children could review social skills in real-life situations. Sauvé et al. (2018) noted that group leaders tailored interventions (e.g., skills to practice at home) to child needs. Parents reported decreases in child anxiety levels and improvement in emotion regulation skills. Some of the children indicated decreases in anxiety, while others did not. Sauvé et al. (2018) concluded that for children who reported anxiety reduction, decreases were clinically significant. Therefore, social skills may help attenuate anxiety symptoms and be a tool, in combination with other interventions (e.g., exposure with rewards), to help children with ASD reduce symptoms of anxiety. On the other hand, many of the children were still experiencing clinically significant anxiety after the intervention had ended. The SAS "detective intervention" was developed for children with Asperger's Disorder or ASD (Beaumont & Sofronoff, 2008) and therefore may be more appropriate for use with youth with higher levels of cognitive functioning.

Beaumont, Rotolone, and Sofronoff (2015) evaluated the impact of the Secret Agent Society after the intervention was delivered in a school setting. The intervention was delivered to children between 7 and 12 years (64 boys and 5 girls). Participants had IQs of 79 or higher, to ensure that they could understand program content. Teachers, special education staff, and school counselors facilitated SAS groups. Facilitators used a manual (revised from Beaumont, 2010) to deliver the SAS training. Children played the computer game to practice social skills at home and recorded their efforts in a diary. For roughly half of the children, facilitators had structured homework requirements to allow children to practice skills. The other half used judgment to incorporate the practice missions in their training. Results showed gains in social skills for both groups. However, in terms of anxiety management, only parents of children who were in the structured homework group showed reductions in children's anxiety. The practice missions or homework assignments were assumed to be successful, because children were showing improved social skills (including managing upset and negative behaviors) and anxiety management at home. Beaumont et al. (2015) concluded that school-based delivery of the program may offer more support for children than use of the intervention in other types of community settings.

Sofronoff, Silva, and Beaumont (2017) conducted another trial of the Secret Agent Society (SAS), in a parent-directed implementation of the activities. Skills taught included recognition of emotions in others, understanding nonverbal behaviors in interactions, and using relaxation strategies to feel calmer and stronger. A thought tracker was used to record negative thoughts. Further, a mindfulness-based approach was used to monitor negative thinking, improve relaxation, and use more positive thoughts. Step-by-step guidelines for introductions, playing with others and coping with mistakes were part of the curriculum. Children also learned to understand teasing and "nasty deeds" and learned "bully guard armor" (plans to prevent and manage bullying). Finally, they also learned ways to cope with uncertainty, should there be a change in routine. And they again found that children participating in this program showed improved social skills and reduced anxiety. Sofronoff et al. (2017) highlighted the use of computer instruction as being critical in teaching skills. Learning ways to use scripts, social stories, and visual cards to script steps of the SAS Program for children with more severe cognitive impairment will be important.

It may be that children with more significant cognitive delays can learn parts of the program or learn the program over a longer period of time (compared to the usual 8- to 10-week implementation period).

Intervention Program: BIACA Program Wood et al. (2015) used a cognitive behavioral therapy (CBT) program with exposure to anxiety-provoking events and stimuli, challenging irrational beliefs, and supportive behaviors of caregivers to assist children with ASD in dealing with anxiety. Their participants were 33 youth with ASD between 11 and 15 years of age. Diagnosis was confirmed using structured interviews with parents and children. Clinicians (psychology students supervised by trained clinicians) used interventions in the *Behavioral Interventions for Anxiety in Children with Autism* (BIACA) Manual developed by Wood, Drahota, Sze, Har, et al. (2009) and Wood, Drahota, Sze, Van Dyke, et al. (2009). This manual capitalizes on a modular approach. Information on coping with anxiety, such as using behavioral activation and cognitive restructuring to reduce negative thoughts and self-talk as well as exposures to feared events and stimuli, were used to help youth reduce anxiety. Clinicians also reviewed social skills for interacting with peers to assist with social anxiety. Parents participated in training as well and learned about improving communication and social skills. Parents learned about home-based exposure (to power through anxiety) and reward systems to use to help reinforce positive coping. Wood et al. (2015) stated that teachers received consultation. Approximately 79% of the group receiving CBT showed improvement in symptoms after treatment compared to about 29% improvement for youth in the waitlist control group. Weaknesses of Wood et al.'s (2015) program were that there was not depth information on parent training for helping youth with social skills or information about the teacher consultations. Having more detail on these interventions might help others seeking to replicate Wood et al.'s (2015) study.

Wood, Drahota, Sze, Har, et al. (2009) provided CBT to 36 youth with ASD between the ages of 7 and 11 years (mean age of about 9 years). They randomly assigned youth to a treatment or control (intent to treat) group. The intervention was delivered by doctoral students in clinical psychology, who were receiving supervision. Children participated in weekly sessions lasting for about 90 min. Children learned about recognizing emotions, how to change negative thinking (e.g., cognitive restructuring), and how to face feared situations. After learning techniques to help face anxiety-provoking situations, children practiced overcoming their fears during vivo exposures. In the exposure sessions they learned to move through their fears, using coping skills to help reduce their anxiety. Clinicians constructed a fear hierarchy, where children listed out their fears and then ranked them from least to most feared situations. Children worked through less feared to more feared situations using coping to remain calm through each situation. Children were rewarded as they moved through fears and tackled those that were higher (related to having higher levels of anxiety) on their hierarchies.

Parent training featured learning to support children during exposure to feared situations and use positive reinforcement when children dealt with fears (Wood, Drahota, Sze, Har, et al., 2009). Parents learned to use communication skills with children to promote their independence in completing daily living tasks (e.g., dressing and self-help skills). Moreover, children and parents learned social skills, such as giving complements, being a good sport, and appropriate ways to engage in interactions with others. Children were assigned peer buddies at school. The intervention program was flexible, and clinicians could select training modules that were appropriate for the child's needs. Findings suggested that children were able to begin to move through feared events and situations. Results indicated parents reported decreased anxiety for children. A 3-month follow-up indicated that 80% of the children were diagnosis-free. However, child reports did not indicate lower anxiety. It may be that the interventions improved avoidance, but the children were still experiencing fear and worry. Wood, Drahota, Sze, Van Dyke, et al. (2009) presented information about symptoms related to ASD in a second paper. Their findings indicated that symptoms of ASD decreased in the treatment group. They concluded that social communication skills were, in particular, positively impacted by the intervention.

Special Considerations about Social Skills Training Based on their review of literature on social skills training, Rumney and Macmahon (2017) concluded that there is evidence that social skills interventions may help to reduce anxiety, although evidence is not uniformly positive. Research with younger children will advance knowledge in the field. Beaumont and Sofronoff's (2008) SAS training has been implemented with elementary school-age children, and positive results show promise for the future. Most interventions are complex treatment packages and whether one or two components of the package are responsible for change is unknown. That is, we do not know the relative contributions of the different components of the treatment packages (e.g., education, exposure, skills training). Understanding how and why social skills interventions work will provide information about whether the "skills-building" makes the difference or exposure to social situations through practice and homework is what is helping youth. Rumney and Macmahon (2017) concluded that parent training was critical to the success of social skills interventions. More research, with parents as coaches and trainers, is needed to determine how parents make interventions work at home.

Anxiety may increase in children with ASD who have higher intellectual or cognitive functioning and it may increase with age (van Steensel & Heeman, 2017). Older youth may be more aware of their social skills deficits, contributing to their anxiety. Clinicians need to be assessing anxiety as children age to be able to design developmentally appropriate interventions. Including social skills interventions in therapy (e.g., Wood et al., 2015) may provide adolescents with a "refresher" in terms of social skills training and allow them to discuss new social issues that may be a source of anxiety. As mentioned, information about treatments for youth with relatively lower cognitive functioning (IQs below 70) is needed, to determine how to reduce fears for this group. Children with relatively lower cognitive functioning may experience fear related to changes in routine or related to interruption of repetitive behaviors. Learning breathing skills and being able to take a break and take some breaths may be a possible calming strategy. Graded exposures with edible reinforcers could potentially help them be less avoidant, and perhaps less fearful, when routines change.

Two Case Studies

Case 1: Phobia Related to Storms DJ was a 12-year-old boy with ASD and anxiety. He was high functioning and attended school with the help of an assistant. He was particularly anxious during storms. There had been a significant storm (e.g., hurricane level), and DJ was home during the storm. A window broke and sirens sounded, with the family retiring to the basement. His parents requested treatment for his fear of storms. Therapy began by understanding his fears and fear behaviors. DJ began crying when rain began, and then he asked to go to his room. He yelled, cried, flapped his hands, and rocked when it rained hard or there was thunder and lightning. It was difficult to develop a fear hierarchy, but sounds were triggers for anxious behaviors (rocking and flapping his hands, with hand-flapping occurring as anxiety increased). DJ really enjoyed chocolate as a reward. DJ's parents agreed that chocolate would be acceptable to use as a reward for positive coping.

The therapist taught DJ to use breathing to relax. DJ was able to smell a flower and blow out a birthday candle (repeating this five times) to help himself relax. DJ and the therapist talked about how he would need to be able to cope with noise and lightning associated with storms, which were a part of nature. He practiced listening to storms on the iPad during sessions (breathing first), then turning on the iPad, listening for a bit, and turning it off. After this, he received some chocolate and was praised for coping with his fear of storms. The storms and rain noise selected on the iPad was presented in a hierarchy from slow and relatively noiseless (calm rain) for 1 min to louder rain for 5 min over a series of sessions. The therapist increased the loud rain "listening" to 8 min and DJ was still successful. Next, listening to louder storms with mild thunder was added and DJ learned to listen without becoming upset. His parents practiced with him as he listened to the iPad at home. They were able to increase DJ's ability to listen to storms to over 10 min.

Next, DJ's parents brought him when a storm was beginning. DJ enjoyed tossing a ball with his dad. Thus, this activity was begun as the storm began. He and his dad tossed the ball as the sky darkened and a storm came. He received chocolate from the therapist after every five throws. He practiced his calming breaths before he threw balls back to his Dad. After the storm began in earnest, the therapist, DJ's parents, and DJ went inside. They watched the storm from inside and talked about being safe indoors. DJ received chocolate periodically, if he was not rocking, hand flapping, or talking loudly and if he was practicing his calming breaths. He received lots of praise from his parents and "high fives" (something DJ enjoyed) for his good coping. After this session, DJ's parents were instructed to repeat the activities at home, with tossing a bean bag in the house as an alternative, if a game of catch was not appropriate. His parents did this on two more occasions.

As a next step, DJ's parents began fading the use of chocolate to receiving it every 15 min, and then moved to providing a piece of candy at the end of the storm, if DJ had coped without rocking, hand-flapping, and/or yelling. DJ's parents reported that the intervention was a positive one. After practicing over the summer, they felt that he was no longer severely afraid of storms. Upon receiving parental consent, the therapist shared the intervention with DJ's teacher and staff at the center where he participated in social skills training. His parents and teacher did not follow up to inform the therapist about whether the intervention was implemented at school. His parents and DJ did not return for treatment after DJ's behavior had improved. They did continue treatment at a local center for youth with ASD where they had access to support groups and a full continuum of services for youth with ASD.

Case 2: Anxiety about Social Interactions Jackson was 14 years of age, and he was experiencing anxiety related to social skills deficits. Specifically, free time in the classroom was very frustrating. Observational data revealed that when Jackson was able to work alone, with his tablet, his behavior was calm during free time. When he did not have his tablet and was asked to interact with peers (board games or making crafts), he became very anxious and began to bite his left hand between his thumb and index finger. Jackson had a very significant callus in this area, and his repeated biting could cause it to bleed. Infection in the area was a concern. Teacher and parent report and observational data revealed that Jackson did not have skills for conversing with peers or was not willing to display his skills. He greatly valued time on his tablet to play games.

In order to develop an initial treatment for Jackson's anxiety, a three-part intervention was developed. First, Jackson was taught social scripts for interacting over board games during free play. Second, his social skills steps were outlined with picture cues on an "interaction card." Third, he was told that if he used the skills and played a board game during the first 10 min of free time, then he could play on his tablet for the final 5 min of free time. Fourth, teachers reduced Jackson's solitary play time and began encouraging Jackson to play one board game (the game involved counting, an area of strength for Jackson) with one person during free play periods. Data on hand-biting was recorded during free time as well as information on involvement with peers. Results for the first month of the intervention indicated reduced hand-biting (reduced 30% from baseline levels) and increased time with one peer. For the intervention to work, a teacher's aide had to initiate invitations to play the game. A subsequent step to add to the interaction card might be to ask a peer to play a game or accepting an invitation to play a game.

This case study was an AB design. Hence, there are limitations, in terms of discussing effectiveness of the intervention, in comparison to a more thorough ABAB (multiple baseline design; see Kennedy, 2005). Given the atypical anxiety displayed by many children with autism (Kerns et al., 2014), and given the value of case studies in this field (Odom et al., 2003), the ABAB design may not be used. It may not be ethical or advisable to withdraw a successful treatment, especially if the child has been engaging in self-injurious behavior(s). Teachers and Jackson's parents were very pleased with the intervention. They felt that Jackson was less anxious and he benefitted from having a structured role and behavioral cues for appropriate social actions during a social situation. In this case, visual strategies showed steps in the interaction and were a communication tool (Hodgdon, 1999), providing a guide for social interaction that could reduce anxiety for Jackson.

If a clinician wanted to involve Jackson in other activities, he or she might first review Jackson's role in the activities and then develop social scripts, describing social behaviors Jackson could use across activities. After this, a next step might be determining Jackson's activity preferences, so that additional social activities could be designed around his interests. After practicing his role and social responses in each activity, Jackson could receive an activity schedule, which would be an interaction card (with visual cues) letting him know what activities he could try. The interaction card could depict specific instructions about how to engage in the activity. Role play and demonstrations could be used to teach Jackson how to use the interaction card. McClannahan and Krantz (2010) provide guidance for developing visually based activity schedules. Another "change" that may spark anxiety in children with autism is transitions between classrooms. Pierce, Spriggs, Gast, and Luscre (2013) reported that visual schedules, depicting what to do and what is happening next, can aide children with ASD in transitioning. As mentioned, visual scripts and activity schedules may be more effective if paired with reinforcement, such as engaging in a preferred activity (Waters et al., 2009). Token systems could be used to develop a reinforcement system, as tackling social abilities and ability to cope with changes may be long-term interventions for some individuals with ASD.

Conclusions

This chapter presents information about treating anxiety in children and adolescents with ASD. Use of graded exposure, moving from less feared to most feared situations, may be a successful intervention for treating anxiety. Rewards for working through anxiety and facing fears, at each step in the fear hierarchy or graded exposure experience, may be necessary. Involving parents and teachers in treatment and teaching them to use reinforcers and how to support their children with calming techniques is a vital part of treatment. Several of the interventions (e.g., Wood, Drahota, Sze, Har, et al., 2009) also used social skills interventions to target communication and social interaction deficits that are related to anxiety in children with ASD. Moreover, some youth with ASD can have a negative cognitive set or talk negatively to themselves. Teaching positive and self-encouraging statements may be an intervention to use with some children and adolescents, particularly those who are higher functioning (van Steensel & Heeman, 2017). Future research is needed to determine if youth with ASD process threatening stimuli differently compared to youth who are developing typically (Ozsivadjian et al., 2012). For example, do children with ASD have memory biases or problems that alter their processing of threat information? Finding out about biases may lead to the development of different interventions that may improve skills and thereby decrease feelings of anxiety. Finally, future studies should examine whether current interventions work with children who are not high functioning. Modifying interventions for children who are not high functioning will be another valuable contribution to existing literature.

References

American Psychiatric Association (DSM). (2013). *Diagnostic and statistical manual of mental disorders* (5th ed.). Washington, DC: Author.

Beaumont, R. (2010). *Secret Agent Society: Solving the mystery of social encounters—facilitator kits*. Milton, Australia: The Social Skills Training Institute.

Beaumont, R., Rotolone, C., & Sofronoff, K. (2015). The Secret Agent Society Social Skills Program for children with high-functioning Autism Spectrum Disorders: A comparison of two school variants. *Psychology in the Schools, 52*(4), 390–402. https://doi.org/10.1002/pits.21831

Beaumont, R., & Sofronoff, K. (2008). A multi-component social skills intervention for children with Asperger syndrome: The junior detective training program. *Journal of Child Psychology and Psychiatry, 49*(7), 743–753. https://doi.org/10.1111/j.1469-7610.2008.01920.x

Black, K. R., Stevenson, R. A., Segers, M., Ncube, B. L., Sun, S. Z., Phillip-Muller, A., … Ferber, S. (2017). Linking anxiety and insistence on sameness in autistic children: The role of sensory hypersensitivity. *Journal of Autism and Development Disorders, 47*(8), 2459–2470. https://doi.org/10.1007/s10803-017-3161-x

Caron, C., & Rutter, M. (1991). Comorbidity in child psychopathology: Concepts, issues, and research strategies. *Journal of Child Psychology and Psychiatry & Allied Disciplines, 32*(7), 1063–1080. https://doi.org/10.1111/j1469-7610.1991.tb00350x

Cho, S., Noor, N. H. B. M., & Sonoyama, S. (2017). A review of activity schedules for individuals with Autism Spectrum Disorder. *Journal of Special Education Research, 5*(2), 65–76. https://doi.org/10.6033/specialeducation.5.65

Cunningham, A. B., & Schreibman, L. (2008). Stereotypy in autism: The importance of function. *Research in Autism Spectrum Disorders, 2*(3), 469–479. https://doi.org/10.1016/j.rasd.2007.09.006

Gotham, K., Bishop, S. L., Hus, V., Huerta, M., Lund, S., Buja, A., … Lord, C. (2013). Exploring the relationship between anxiety and insistence on sameness in autism spectrum disorders. *Autism Research, 6*(1), 33–41. https://doi.org/10.1002/aur.1263

Gresham, F. M., Watson, T. S., & Skinner, C. H. (2001). Functional behavioral assessment: Principles, procedures, and future directions. *School Psychology Review, 30*(2), 156–172.

Hodgdon, L. A. (1999). *Solving behavior problems in Autism: Improving communication with visual strategies*. Troy, MI: Quirk Roberts Publishing.

Kennedy, C. H. (2005). *Single-case designs for educational research*. Boston: Pearson.

Kerns, C. M., & Kendall, P. C. (2012). The presentation and classification of anxiety in autism spectrum disorder. *Clinical Psychology Science and Practice, 19*(4), 323–347. https://doi.org/10.1111/cpsp.12009

Kerns, C. M., Kendall, P. C., Berry, L., Souders, M. C., Franklin, M. E., Schultz, R. T., … Herrington, J. (2014). Traditional and atypical presentations of anxiety in youth with autism spectrum disorder. *Journal of Autism and Developmental Disorders, 44*(11), 2851–2861. https://doi.org/10.1007/s10803-014-2141-7

Knight, V., Sartini, E., & Spriggs, A. D. (2015). Evaluating visual activity schedules as evidence-based practice for individuals with autism spectrum disorders. *Journal of Autism and Developmental Disorders, 45*, 157–178. https://doi.org/10.1007/s10803-014-2201-z

Kulage, K. M., Smaldone, A. M., & Cohn, E. G. (2014). How will DSM-5 affect autism diagnosis? A systematic literature review and meta-analysis. *Journal of Autism and Developmental Disorders, 44*(8), 1918–1932. https://doi.org/10.1007/s10803-014-2065-2

Lane, S. J., Reynolds, S., & Dumenci, L. (2012). Sensory oversensitivity and anxiety in typically developing children and children with Autism and Attention Deficit Hyperactivity Disorder: Cause or coexistence? *American Journal of Occupational Therapy, 66*, 595–603. https://doi.org/10.5014/ajot.2012.004523

McClannahan, L. E., & Krantz, P. J. (2010). *Activity schedules for children with autism: Teaching independent behavior*. Bethesda, MD: Woodbine House.

Mesibov, G. B., Browder, D. M., & Kirkland, C. (2002). Using individualized schedules as a component of positive behavioral support for students with developmental disabilities. *Journal of Positive Behavior Interventions, 4*, 73–79. https://doi.org/10.1177/109830070200400202

Mesibov, G. B., & Shea, V. (2010). The TEACCH Program in the era of evidence-based practice. *Journal of Autism and Developmental Disorders, 40*, 570–579. https://doi.org/10.1007/s10803-009-0901-6

Odom, S. L., Brown, W. H., Frey, T., Karasu, N., Smith-Canter, L. L., & Strain, P. S. (2003). Evidence-based practices for young children with autism: Contributions for single-subject design research. *Focus on Autism and Other Developmental Disabilities, 18*(3), 166–175.

Ozsivadjian, A., Knott, F., & Magiati, I. (2012). Parent and child perspectives on the nature of anxiety in children and young people with autism spectrum disorders: A focus group study. *Autism, 16*(2), 107–121. https://doi.org/10.1177/1362361311431703

Pierce, J. M., Spriggs, A. D., Gast, D. L., & Luscre, D. (2013). Effects of visual activity schedules on independent classroom transitions for students with autism. *International Journal of Disability, Development and Education, 60*(3), 253–269. https://doi.org/10.1080/1034912X.2013.812191

Rumney, H., & Macmahon, K. (2017). Do social skills interventions positively influence mood in children and young people with autism? A systematic review. *Mental Health & Prevention, 5*, 12–20. https://doi.org/10.1016/j.mhp.2016.12.001

Sauvé, J. S., O'Haire, C., Hall, H., Lane, C., & Hudson, B. O. (2018). Adapting a social skills intervention for children with Autism within an urban specialty community clinic. *Evidence-Based Practice in Child and Adolescent Mental Health, 3*(4), 219–235. https://doi.org/10.1080/23794925.2018.1483214

Sofronoff, K., Silva, J., & Beaumont, R. (2017). The Secret Agent Society Social-Emotional Skills Program for children with high-functioning Autism Spectrum Disorder: A parent-directed trial. *Focus on Autism and Other Developmental Disabilities, 32*(1), 55–70. https://doi.org/10.1177/1088357615583467

Sukhodolsky, D. G., Bloch, M. H., Panza, K. E., & Reichow, B. (2013). Cognitive behavioral therapy for anxiety in children with high-functioning Autism: A meta-analysis. *Pediatrics, 132*, e1341–e1350. https://doi.org/10.1542/pens.2013-1193

van Steensel, F., & Heeman, E. J. (2017). Anxiety levels in children with Autism Spectrum Disorder: A meta-analysis. *Journal of Child and Family Studies, 26*(7), 1753–1767. https://doi.org/10.1007/s10826-017-0687-7

van Steensel, F. J., Bögels, S. M., & Perrin, S. (2011). Anxiety disorders in children and adolescents with autistic spectrum disorders: A meta-analysis. *Clinical Child and Family Psychology Review, 14*(3), 302–317. https://doi.org/10.1007/s10567-011-0097-0

Vasa, R. A., & Masurek, M. O. (2015). An update on anxiety in youth with autism spectrum disorders. *Current Opinions in Psychiatry, 28*(2), 83–90. https://doi.org/10.1097/YCO.0000000000000133

Volkmar, F., Siegel, M., Woodbury-Smith, M., King, B., McCracken, J., & State, M. (2014). Practice parameter for the assessment and treatment of children and adolescents with autism spectrum disorder. *Journal of the American Academy of Child & Adolescent Psychiatry, 53*(2), 237–257. https://doi.org/10.1016/j.jaac.2013.10.013

Waters, M. B., Lerman, D. C., & Hovanetz, A. N. (2009). Separate and combined effects of visual schedules and extinction plus differential reinforcement on problem behavior occasioned by transitions. *Journal of Applied Behavior Analysis, 42*(2), 309–313. https://doi.org/10.1091/jaba.2009.42-309

White, S. W., Lerner, M. D., McLeod, B. D., Wood, J. J., Ginsburg, G. S., Kerns, C., … Compton, S. (2015). Anxiety in youth with and without autism spectrum disorder: Examination of factorial equivalence. *Behavior Therapy, 46*(1), 40–53. https://doi.org/10.1016/j.beth.2014.05.005

Wood, J. J., Drahota, A., Sze, K., Har, K., Chou, A., & Langer, D. A. (2009). Cognitive behavioral therapy for anxiety in children with autism spectrum disorders: A randomized controlled trial. *Journal of Child Psychology and Psychiatry, 50*(3), 224–234. https://doi.org/10.1111/j.1469-7610.2008.01948.x

Wood, J. J., Drahota, A., Sze, K., Van Dyke, M., Decker, K., Fujii, C., … Spiker, M. (2009). Brief Report: Effects of cognitive behavior therapy on parent reported Autism symptoms in school-age children with high-functioning autism. *Journal of Autism and Developmental Disorders, 39*, 1608–1612. https://doi.org/10.1007/s10803-009-0791-7

Wood, J. J., Ehrenreich-May, J., Alessandri, M., Fujii, C., Renno, P., Laugeson, E., … Storch, E. (2015). Cognitive behavioral therapy for early adolescents with Autism Spectrum Disorders and clinical anxiety: A randomized, controlled trial. *Behavior Therapy, 46*, 7–19. https://doi.org/10.1016/j.beth.2014.01.002

Chapter 6
Chronic Illness and Anxiety in Children

Introduction

Children with chronic illnesses may have more difficulties with emotional and behavioral functioning compared to children who do not face illnesses (Blackman, Gurka, Gurka, & Oliver, 2011; Compas, Jaser, Dunn, & Rodriguez, 2012). The overall rate of emotional and behavioral problems in children with chronic illnesses is estimated at 15%, and this is a higher rate of problems compared to children in the general population (Ferro & Boyle, 2015). Children with chronic illnesses may have more internalizing problems, such as anxiety (Pinquart & Shen, 2011). Ferro and Boyle (2015) assessed emotional functioning in children ages 10–15 years, with a variety of chronic illnesses, and found that children with this age range had higher risk for anxiety and depression than their counterparts who did not have chronic illnesses.

Blackman et al. (2011) used a national sample and compared anxiety and depression to "acting out" or externalizing problems (e.g., acting out, arguing, bullying) for children with chronic illnesses, including headaches, arthritis/joint problems, diabetes, blood disorders (e.g., sickle cell disease), and heart problems. They found that internalizing and externalizing problems may occur at different rates for different health problems. For instance, they found higher rates of anxiety and depression for children with headaches, arthritis/joint problems, and diabetes. However, rates internalizing and externalizing problems were roughly equivalent for children who had blood disorders and heart problems. Interestingly, they reported that Attention-Deficit Hyperactivity Disorder was higher than average (twice as high) for children with chronic conditions (Blackman et al., 2011).

Blackman et al. (2011) mentioned that concern for children with chronic illnesses increases as they grow older, as there may be cumulative effects of the condition and higher emotional demands, which, in turn, may exacerbate mental health problems. They added that boys may experience emotional upset if they have slow

L. Nabors, *Anxiety Management in Children with Mental and Physical Health Problems*, Springer Series on Child and Family Studies,
https://doi.org/10.1007/978-3-030-35606-4_6

growth and physical development in adolescence, which can be a factor with some illnesses. Blackman et al. (2011) did not find a relationship between pain and emotional functioning. On the other hand, Blackman et al. (2011) highlighted the fact that other researchers have discovered a relationship between pain, depression, and anxiety for children who have chronic illnesses.

Anxiety and Chronic Illnesses Other researchers have studied anxiety for children with specific chronic illnesses. For example, Dudeney, Sharpe, Jaffe, Jones, and Hunt (2017) conducted a meta-analysis to improve knowledge of anxiety for youth with asthma. They reported a "... prevalence rate of 22.7% [which was] ... more than three times higher than the prevalence in healthy youth" (Dudeney et al., 2017, p. 1). Their prevalence rate was based on 15 studies included in their meta-analysis (n = 7443). Youth demonstrated a "spread" of different types of anxiety disorders (p. 6), including separation anxiety, social phobia, Generalized Anxiety Disorder (GAD), agoraphobia, and Panic Disorder. Rates of GAD and social phobia were particularly high. Fidler et al. (2019) also found that youth with anxiety were likely to endorse symptoms of GAD. Researchers have recommended that health professionals use screening tools and questions to identify anxiety in children with asthma so that appropriate referral for counseling can be provided when indicated (Dudeney et al., 2017; Fidler et al., 2019). Asking children if they have worries that cause them to avoid situations and make them upset often, and asking them if their worries interfere with their daily functioning are initial screening questions. Asking children if they have worries about their illness and asking if they would like to speak to a professional, are general questions to determine if a referral to a pediatric psychologist is needed.

Quittner et al. (2016; for the International Committee on Mental Health in Cystic Fibrosis) wrote a paper on psychological distress in individuals with Cystic Fibrosis (CF). They concluded that individuals with CF face significant anxiety and deal with significant levels of procedural anxiety. They defined procedural anxiety as, "... an acute and excessive fear of a medical or surgical procedure that results in stress or avoidance" (p. 27). Anxiety, along with depression, was elevated in youth with CF. Negative emotional symptoms were related to symptom severity, poorer lung functioning, and more frequent hospitalizations. Quittner et al. (2016) mentioned that the painful procedures, including blood draws, intravenous lines, and catheter insertions were a source of worry and fear. They recommended screening for psychological symptoms and referral for therapy for mental health problems. Additionally, they suggested training in cognitive-behavioral skills and problem-solving to assist patients with CF in coping with anxiety. If anxiety related to medical procedures did not respond to cognitive-behavioral techniques (e.g., relaxation, imagery), they recommended that medications (e.g., benzodiazepine) be considered for short-term use. Additional patient monitoring to protect the patient from abuse might be indicated should a medication trial be implemented. Quittner et al. (2016) called for more research with patients who had CF so that mental health interventions could be tailored to their concerns.

Similarly, Reigada et al. (2013) reported that children and adolescents who were diagnosed with Crohn's disease were likely to experience anxiety. Symptoms children with Crohn's disease may face, among a host of other symptoms, are stomach aches/abdominal pain, diarrhea, abdominal mass, and extraintestinal symptoms (e.g., abscesses, fissure). These researchers examined anxiety using the *Screen for Child Anxiety Related Disorders* or *SCARED* measure (Birmaher et al., 1999). This is appropriate for children and adolescents aged nine to 18 years. The survey consists of 41 items, which may be overwhelming for some youth. However, there are some very helpful questions, such as assessment of physiological symptoms (e.g., when scared it is hard to breathe), excessive fear (e.g., when frightened it feels like I am going crazy), and how anxiety can limit life opportunities (e.g., I worry about going to school, worry about life not working out for me). Reigada et al. (2013) reported that youth with Crohn's disease who were experiencing moderate-to-severe symptoms were more likely to experience anxiety. Fifty percent of the children in their sample reported anxiety in a specific area on the *SCARED*, such as school, general worries, or separation anxiety. Reigada et al. (2013) mentioned that anxiety can potentially increase children's sensitivity to gastrointestinal symptoms, creating a vicious cycle. More study of this potential cycle, and the role health professionals can play in alleviating it, will provide direction for management of anxiety for children with this difficult disorder.

Knight et al. (2015) examined risk factors related to anxiety (and depression) in children with lupus (systemic lupus erythematosus; SLE), mixed connective tissue disease, and children with diabetes. Their "interest group" was children with SLE and mixed connective tissue disease. Their comparison group was children with diabetes and a comparison group of healthy children. They used the *SCARED* (Birmaher et al., 1997) to assess child anxiety. Anxiety levels were at 30% for the children with chronic illnesses, which was higher than anxiety levels in children who did not have chronic illnesses. As mentioned, they assessed depression, which was common. Furthermore, depression was higher in children of color. They highlighted the need to screen for mental health concerns in youth with chronic illnesses as being foundational to a "whole child" approach for child wellness. Referral for treatment, when youth experience either depression or anxiety, can potentially mitigate difficulties and decrease chances of poor psychosocial outcomes for youth (Knight et al., 2015).

Somatic Complaints and Anxiety Children with anxiety can report a high number of somatic complaints. Crawley et al. (2014) examined somatic symptoms in a sample of over 450 youth, ages 7–17 years, with anxiety disorders, namely, GAD, separation anxiety disorder, and social phobia. Children rated their physical symptoms and their severity on a checklist. Children with anxiety often reported headaches and stomach aches, head colds or sniffles, and sleeping difficulties. It is noteworthy that the number of physical symptoms decreased over treatment, which featured cognitive-behavioral therapy, sertraline, a combination of treatments, or a placebo pill. Interestingly, physical symptoms decreased in youth who took a placebo pill. Crawley et al. (2014) speculated that perhaps youth with anxiety are "hyperaware" of their physical state, and this may be a reason for paying more attention to physical symptoms. If children thought their symptoms would improve, perhaps it would cause a difference in hyperawareness (i.e., causing success in the placebo condition). Crawley et al. (2014) remarked that older youth may have more physical symptoms or may notice them more, and further research will be needed to understand the nature and impact of physical symptoms for older youth.

Strategies for Anxiety Management

Children with chronic illnesses can face significant anxiety related to undergoing medical procedures (Compas et al., 2012; Pinquart & Shen, 2011). Implementation of cognitive-behavioral strategies may reduce anxiety during hospitalization and medical procedures (Pao & Bosk, 2011; Uman, Chambers, McGrath, & Kisely, 2008). Children with illnesses may need to develop personalized anxiety management strategies to help them cope with their unique situations. Kendall, Settipani, and Cummings (2012) recommended personalizing successful CBT strategies to help children cope with anxiety, and this practice may be especially helpful for children with chronic illnesses. Nabors, Odar Stough, Combs, and Elkins (2019) worked with children to help them turn cognitive-behavioral strategies into a personalized coping menu. This menu had strategies to help children deal with worries related to their chronic illnesses. An example of a menu is presented in Fig. 6.1.

Nabors, Odar Stough, et al. (2019) used strategies presented in the "*Coping Positively with My Worries Manual for Kids: Getting off the Worry RaceTrack!*" developed by Nabors and Elkins (2017) to teach children and parents an anxiety management intervention. Strategies in this manual included relaxation (breathing and muscle relaxation), imagery (going to the beach or a favorite place), receiving support from a loved one, and using distraction (through play and doing fun things). Support from parents and family also was a coping tool. Nabors and Elkins (2017) used a noncategorical approach (Stein & Jessop, 1982) to develop a generalized manual so that strategies would work for children coping with a variety of different illnesses. The menu allowed children to personalize strategies.

For older youth, a coping menu might not be developmentally appropriate. Adolescents can review strategies and make a table, perhaps on a notecard, to record which strategies they will use to cope with their medically-related worries. Figure 6.2 presents a sample table that might be helpful for older youth to use to document their ideas for personalizing anxiety management strategies (Kendall et al., 2012). This will provide them with a record of what they will use and when.

Others have determined that relaxation, distraction, and reinforcement of coping behaviors are positive strategies for children who face medical fears. Researchers have found that breathing deeply or diaphragmatic breathing; distraction (e.g., play, games, or positive imagery); muscle relaxation; and reinforcement of positive coping responses are strategies that work for children (Koller & Goldman, 2012; Uman et al., 2008). Li, Chung, Ho, and Kwok (2016) reported that toy play can serve as a

Coping Menu for My Coping Restaurant

My worry triggers: ____

**Choose a strategy to help you deal with your worry!*

Breakfast (Distraction) 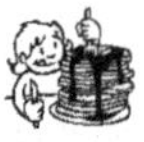

- ❖ Do my favorite activity (color, read, movie, puzzle) ____________________
- ❖ Play with my calming toy ______________________________________
- ❖ Talk to an adult or a friend _____________________________________

Lunch (Imagination) 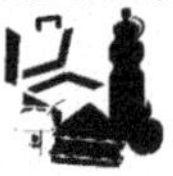

- ❖ Imagine my happy place ______________________________________
- ❖ Be my own superhero ____

Dinner (Relaxation) 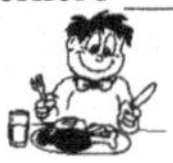

- ❖ Rock Sponge Technique. I will do this _______ times
- ❖ Focus on my breathing – Blow up ______ beach balls in my belly

Dessert (Positive Self Talk/Think) 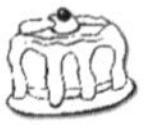

- ❖ Think happy thoughts
- ❖ Say positive things to myself ____________________________________

How will you reward yourself for dealing with your worries? ________________________

Fig. 6.1 Sample items from a children's coping menu

distraction technique, resulting in decreases in negative emotion and behavior, reduced anxiety, and reduced pain during hospitalizations. Patel et al. (2006) found that when children played video games they did not report increased anxiety during an anesthesia induction. Distraction is a key strategy when children are coping with painful procedures (Compas et al., 2012; Dahlquist et al., 2002), and this was the case for many of the children in the study conducted by Nabors, Odar Stough, et al. (2019). Additionally, Nabors, Odar Stough, et al. (2019) found the chief worry mentioned by children was fear of invasive procedures with needles, followed by general references to surgery and medical procedures. Play was another critical distraction strategy for children in the aforementioned study. Others have found that play with games was a critical distraction tool for children (e.g., Patel et al., 2006). Nabors, Odar Stough, et al. (2019) found that younger children distracted themselves with favorite stuffed animals and blankets (which were considered to be "calming objects"), while older children preferred electronics for distraction. Music and art were other key distraction tools used by children, who really appreciated help and support from Child Life specialists during hospitalization.

Instructions What strategies will you use to get your mind off your worries? Will it be Positive Talk? Relaxation? Or maybe Distraction by doing something fun? How about going to your favorite place in your imagination? When will you use your strategy? Always tell yourself great job after you use a strategy. Record your strategies in the boxes below. Write (or have your parent write) when you can use each strategy.		
Name of Strategy	When I can use it	Say "Good Job" to myself

Fig. 6.2 Table for personalizing anxiety strategies for older youth

Researchers have used treatment "packages" consisting of several CBT interventions to help children with chronic illnesses. For instance, Reigada et al. (2013) developed an intervention to help children with Inflammatory Bowel Disease (IBD). They used relaxation, cognitive restructuring (thinking about positive outcomes), and exposure to reduce anxiety for youth. Stapersma et al. (2018) implemented education, cognitive-behavioral strategies, and social skills training for children with IBD. They found improvements in anxiety and depression. Peterson and Shigetomi (1981) found that teaching children (2–10 years) muscle relaxation, distracting mental imagery, and positive self-talk resulted in lower levels of distress experienced by youth during a tonsillectomy. Similarly, Nabors, Odar Stough, et al. (2019) reported that children reported going to the beach or theme parks (riding roller-coasters, etc.) as imaginal strategies, which served to distract them during painful procedures. Younger children used superheroes (e.g., "Wonderwoman," "Thor," "Rainbow Glitter Girl," and "Iron Man") to help them fight their pain and worry, chiefly during invasive procedures. In terms of positive self-talk, children reported repeating "psych up" phrases like, "I can do this. I am brave." These repetitive phrases, almost like mantras, could assist children in coping with hospital- and illness-related worries (Nabors, Odar Stough, et al., 2019).

Parents: A Critical Role

Parents can play a critical role in problem-solving, by helping children select strategies and then implement them during medical procedures (McCarthy & Kleiber, 2006; Peterson & Shigetomi, 1981). Moreover, parents can reinforce their child for coping with his or her worries (Nabors, Odar Stough, et al., 2019). Parents can help their child review coping strategies, and this can provide them with a role as coaches. This may improve their sense of place and give them a purpose as their child undergoes traumatic experiences. Parents also serve as emotional supports for children (Ferro & Boyle, 2015; Nabors, Liddle, Graves, Kamphaus, & Elkins, 2019). Eccleston, Fisher, Law, Bartlett, and Palermo (2015) published a Cochrane review of psychological interventions for parents of youth with chronic illnesses. They reviewed 47 randomized controlled trials. Findings indicated that interventions with parents resulted in more adaptive parenting and parents who employed CBT could help children reduce negative chronic illness symptoms, such as anxiety responses. Moreover, being able to participate and trying to help their child could result in improved mental health of parents (Eccleston et al., 2015). Anthony, Gil, and Schanberg (2003) proposed that parents of children with chronic illnesses can feel worried about their child's future, leading them to consider their children as vulnerable, possibly overprotecting them. This overprotectiveness and concern about further illness episodes may contribute to child anxiety, when parents inadvertently accommodate and reinforce child anxiety. Providing parents with a role that empowers them may reduce parents' worries and, concurrently, alleviate the negative impact of parental worry on child anxiety.

Using similar reasoning, Mullins et al. (2015) noted that uncertainty related to chronic illnesses, such as cancer, can cause stress in parents. Ultimately, parent stress may be related to emotional and behavioral difficulties exhibited by children. Mullins et al. (2015) and Anthony et al. (2003) recommended that clinicians assess parent responses and feelings in order to support them. Helping parents recognize how their perceptions of their child's illness can impact their child may help parents appreciate the power of their views and actions on their child's coping. Mullins et al. (2015) conducted an intervention to teach parents about how illness uncertainty can affect them and help parents increase their own social support. Similarly, Ferro and Boyle (2015) highlighted the importance of improving family support as a means to help both the parents and children cope, thereby reducing worries. Ferro and Boyle (2015) wrote that maternal mood directly impacts children and this should be discussed with mothers. Mullins et al. (2015) recommended teaching parents coping and problem-solving behaviors. Providing parents with a positive coaching role, where they see a way to support their child and support success, may provide a positive direction for their role in helping their child (Norman, Silverman, & Lebowitz, 2015). Mullins et al. (2015) taught parents ways to communicate with the medical team—then, they can become educated and learn about the child's regimen. After opening communication, parents may have opportunities to explain their child's emotions to health professionals. Another role for parents is to reinforce their child's accomplishments in school, in the family, and in their lives. As a success coach, parents can work to build their child's self-esteem, which can reduce anxiety as well as depression in children (Ferro & Boyle, 2015).

Morawska, Calam, and Fraser (2015) reported that parents may feel a lack of confidence in helping their child cope with his or her illness. Morawska et al. (2015) viewed parent needs as being similar across different types of health conditions (taking a noncategorical approach; Stein & Jessop, 1982). This allows for development of general principles that could aid parents in caring for their children. Morawska et al. (2015) believed the burden of disease management may fall primarily to parents, and this can include helping children to manage emotional concerns, such as anxiety. Teaching parents problem-solving skills to help children identify anxiety triggers and reduce the magnitude or strength of their anxiety response empowers parents as helpers and coaches. This has the potential to reduce both parent and child anxiety, which can be bidirectional (Morawska et al., 2015). Furthermore, parents can assist by helping the child express his or her feelings. Nabors, Odar Stough, et al. (2019) noted that parents can be translators—teaching the child's medical team about his or her worries.

As mentioned, parents can learn cognitive-behavioral strategies including breathing, relaxation, imagery, and distraction to support their child in coping with worry. Some of the strategies from a manual developed by Nabors and Elkins (2017) are presented in the Appendix of this chapter. Personalizing the strategies, by allowing the child to pick which strategies he or she will use and recording when and how they will be used, may optimize the effectiveness of strategies (Kendall et al., 2012, see Fig. 6.1). Our research indicated that parents believed that distraction (e.g., doing something fun, playing games, using electronics) and relaxation were the most useful anxiety management strategies. Further research is needed to determine whether the strategies are useful in the long term. However, parents viewed the coping manual (Nabors & Elkins, 2017) positively. The techniques were strategies they could use with their child (Nabors, Odar Stough et al. 2019). If parents do not know any strategies and do not understand the significance of helping the child "power through" anxiety, they may inadvertently allow the child to avoid things, like medical procedures, that can cause the child anxiety. There can be a high level of accommodation with pediatric anxiety, and it can be associated with greater feelings of caregiver burden (Norman et al., 2015). It can be very difficult to watch one's child become more distressed, if he or she is avoiding anxiety-provoking stimuli or events. If parents are "armed" with cognitive-behavioral strategies to help their child, and understand the importance of "powering through" anxiety and praising coping, they can play a prominent role in child coping. This will reduce their child's worry and improve their perceptions of being a successful caregiver. Ultimately, this may reduce perceptions of caregiver burden.

Case Study

Drake and Ginsburg (2012) published results of a case study examining cognitive-behavioral treatment of anxiety for chronic pediatric headache for a 10-year-old boy and his family. The boy (Brian) had a history of anxiety and he worried about pleasing others, doing well in school, and never getting in trouble. Brian worried about his performance in sports and other recreational activities (e.g., choir). He worried about something bad happening to his sister. He also experienced distress when his hands were soiled. Brian was enrolled in 8 weeks of treatment where he learned about how anxiety works, such as how anxiety works in the body, what one thinks, and how one can avoid things and inadvertently increase anxiety. During treatment Brian complained of headaches, and it was determined (by a medical team prior to treatment) that his headaches and anxiety were interrelated. Brian's parents had inadvertently accommodated his worries (Norman et al., 2015). Clinicians taught parents about the worry cycle and provided ideas for helping Brian work through his worries. For example, it was explained that "When you avoid doing things because of headaches, you teach yourself that you are incapable of doing things because you are ill and begin to see yourself as 'sick and helpless.'" (p. 586). Parents were taught to use reinforcement (e.g., praise, rewards) to increase the frequency of "… well and brave behaviors" (p. 587).

Situations causing headache and anxiety were identified and the level of difficulty or worry associated with each situation was determined (e.g., an anxiety hierarchy was developed and worked through in a relaxed state). Brian learned relaxation, tensing muscle groups and releasing them from head to toe (Drake & Ginsburg, 2012). Brian learned cognitive restructuring, to reduce negative self-talk (I can't go to the party because it will be too loud), and to challenge negative thoughts (or distorted thoughts) and replace them with positive ones (I'll try to stay at the party). Brian learned to question his ideas that outcomes would always be negative and think about positive outcomes. A diary was used to record reductions in anxiety. Over time, results were very positive.

In terms of hand-washing due to soiling, Brian worked to delay washing his hands when he thought they were dirty (Drake & Ginsburg, 2012). Use of hand sanitizer during the day was reduced. His parents made progress in learning to reward coping behavior and ignore avoidance behaviors. The SOLVE problem-solving method was taught to Brian and his parents:

> S = settle down (you can solve problems better calm), O = own the problem (identify what parts of the problem are under your control), L = list possible solutions to the problem, V = vote for a solution to try (consider pros and cons of solutions on list), and E = engage in the best solution and evaluate the outcome" (Drake & Ginsburg, 2012, p. 591)

After Brian and his parents learned skills, sessions were devoted to reviewing lessons, discussing relapse, and learning relapse prevention strategies. Brian and his parents were taught to recognize things that might signal worry was recurring. Clinicians, parents, and Brian discussed ideas for implementing strategies to help Brian in anxiety-producing situations. Throughout this course of treatment, Brian's worry and headaches reduced. Toward the end of treatment, Brian still was experiencing some anxiety related to separating from his mother, and she was supporting or accommodating his anxiety response (paying attention, which was inadvertently reinforcing his anxiety behaviors). His mother and a clinician reviewed ideas for promoting independence. This case was very successful. It has been my experience that shrinking worries and eliminating some of them is a successful course of treatment. It may be that parents need to continue to employ worry management strategies because anxiety will often recur or "pop out" in other areas of life once treatment has ended. For instance, Brian could start worrying about friendships or another issue. In these cases, booster sessions to review strategies and reapply them or apply them in new situations may be warranted.

Conclusions

This chapter reviews anxiety management strategies for children with chronic illnesses. Also, a discussion of how children with anxiety may experience more somatic complaints is presented. Further research will be needed to determine the relations among anxiety and sensitivity to somatic issues. There is a significant literature on pain and anxiety that may provide direction for future research. A detailed review of pain is beyond the scope of this chapter (see Fisher, Heathcote, Eccleston, Simons, & Palermo, 2018, and other articles in volume 43 of the *Journal of Pediatric Psychology* in 2018 for information on pain). Ideas for managing anxiety related to medical procedures are conveyed, with distraction and relaxation being particularly successful interventions (Nabors, Odar Stough, et al., 2019). It will be important to find parents a role in helping their children cope with illness and medical procedures, perhaps involving them as anxiety management coaches, a role that will empower them (Morawska et al., 2015; Mullins et al., 2015). The SOLVE method for problem-solving is a simple method that may provide parents with a model of steps to aid their child in resolving situations that are stressful (Drake & Ginsburg, 2012). Empowering children by teaching them coping skills and steps for assessing their impact may assist them in powering through anxiety and personalizing coping strategies.

Appendix

Excerpts from the Coping Positively with My Worries Manual for Kids (Nabors & Elkins, 2017): Explaining Worries and Three Ways to Deal with Worry (Positive Talk, Relaxation, and Imagery).

Explaining Worries to the Child

What does worry do?

- Worry is a normal part of life.

Everyone worries.

But sometimes, if you think about your worries too much, they can take over and get too big.

Let's pretend you are a race car.

When you let the worries take over, your race car runs in circles around the worry race track over and over and cannot get to the finish line.

It is important to realize when you are thinking of the worries over and over and letting your race car go in circles.

If you have the same worry thought over and over,

If your heart beats fast,

If your breathing gets faster,

If your body starts to feel heavy like a rock,

You might be letting the worries take over and getting your car stuck in circles on the worry racetrack.

Explanation of How Worries Work in One's Body

Worry speeds up the body. You breathe faster and your heart beats quicker. Your mind races and thinks about the worries over and over again. If you think of the worries over and over, they grow. The more the worries grow, the more your body speeds up.

Worries can also make your muscles tighten up. Sometimes, when your muscles tighten up, you feel worse and feel more pain. If you tighten up your body and muscles, shots or needle sticks can hurt more.

It is important to push pause on the worries and relax. When you do this, you can slow your body down. Do your best to relax and try not to worry.

Three Ways to Deal with Worry: Positive Talk, Relaxation, and Imagery

Positive Talk

It is good to use positive talk against the worries so you get your brain off the worry racetrack.

Positive talk mean saying to yourself, "I can deal with this needle stick because I have had them before and it turned out OK" or "I can deal with being in the hospital. I can help the doctors and nurses and talk to my family if I need to cheer up."

Say positive things inside your head, like, "I can deal with this."

Relaxation

Here are two techniques to help you relax. Being a rock then a sponge and focusing on your breathing.

Rock–Sponge Technique

Relax by practicing making muscles tight like a rock and then relaxing like a sponge and taking deep breaths. The sponge squeezes out the worry.

Now, it is your turn practice being the superrelaxation sponge kid. Here is what you do …

Sit in a chair or you can lay in your bed.

Make your muscles tight, like a rock (when you do this, if a part of you hurts, do not make it like a rock! Just do the rock where it does not hurt).

Then, make your muscles loose, like a sponge sinking in to your chair or bed.

Take some deep breaths and close your eyes. Repeat until your mind is not going round and round on the worry racetrack!

Focus on Your Breathing

Focusing on your breathing can take your mind off your worry and get you off the worry racetrack.

Close your eyes.

Breathe in nice and slow. Imagine your tummy is a beach ball and you are slowly filling it with air you breathe in.

Hold the beach ball inside your belly until you count to five on your fingers.

Now, slowly breathe out and imagine the beach ball slowly getting smaller.

How many beach balls will you fill and make smaller to help shrink your worry? I will fill ___________ beach balls.

Using Imagination

Imagining a happy place can help you to take a break from your worries.

Trudy's favorite spot is the beach. She thinks about the beach and the ocean and warm sun when she wants a vacation from her worries. Trudy likes to make sand castles and relax at the beach. She pretends the warm sun makes her worries get small. She sees a boat in the water and the birds flying over the water. She hears the waves as they hit the sand. Can you see the beach? Can you hear the water? Now, is your worry smaller?

Take a vacation from your worry … practice going to your favorite place in your imagination.

What is your favorite place?

What is it like?

What happens there?

What does it sound like?

What do you see?

What are you doing?

What happens next?

Note. The interviewer helps the child imagine his or her happy place (a birthday party, vacation spot). The interviewer helps the child imagine all the details, in a linear fashion (What happens next?). The child is encouraged to see him or herself in the event. Examples of questions are, "What do you see, hear, and feel?"

References

Anthony, K. K., Gil, K. M., & Schanberg, L. (2003). Brief report: Parental perceptions of child vulnerability in children with chronic illness. *Journal of Pediatric Psychology, 28*, 185–190. https://doi.org/10.1093/jpepsy/jsg005

Birmaher, B., Brent, D. A., Chiappetta, L., Bridge, J., Monga, S., & Baugher, M. (1999). Psychometric properties of the *Screen for Child Anxiety Related Emotional Disorders* (*SCARED*): A replication study. *Journal of the American Academy of Child and Adolescent Psychiatry, 38*(10), 1230–1236. https://doi.org/10.1097/00004583-199910000-00011

Birmaher, B., Khetarpal, S., Brent, D., Cully, M., Balach, L., Kaufman, J., & Neer, S. M. (1997). The *Screen for Child Anxiety Related Emotional Disorders* (*SCARED*): Scale construction and psychometric characteristics. *Journal of the American Academy of Child and Adolescent Psychiatry, 36*(4), 545–553. https://doi.org/10.1097/00004583-1997040000-00018

Blackman, J. A., Gurka, M. J., Gurka, K. K., & Oliver, M. N. (2011). Emotional, developmental and behavioural co-morbidities of children with chronic health conditions. *Journal of Paediatrics and Child Health, 47*(10), 742–747. https://doi.org/10.1111/j.1440-1754.2011.02044.x

Compas, B. E., Jaser, S. S., Dunn, M. J., & Rodriguez, E. M. (2012). Coping with chronic illness in childhood and adolescences. *Annual Review of Clinical Psychology, 8*, 455–480. https://doi.org/10.1146/annurev-clinpsy-032511-143108

Crawley, S. A., Caporino, N. E., Birmaher, B., Ginsburg, G., Piacentini, J., Albano, A. M., … Kendall, P. C. (2014). Somatic complaints in anxious youth. *Child Psychiatry and Human Development, 45*(4), 398–407. https://doi.org/10.1007/s10578-013-0410-x

Dahlquist, L. M., Busby, S. M., Slifer, K. J., Tucker, C. L., Eischen, S., Hilley, L., & Sulc, W. (2002). Distraction for children of different ages who undergo repeated needle sticks. *Journal of Pediatric Oncology Nursing, 19*, 22–34. https://doi.org/10.1053/jpon.2002.30009

Drake, K. L., & Ginsburg, G. S. (2012). Family-based cognitive-behavioral treatment of chronic pediatric headache and anxiety disorders: A case study. *Child & Youth Care Forum, 41*, 579–598. https://doi.org/10.1007/s10566-012-9174-x

Dudeney, J., Sharpe, L., Jaffe, A., Jones, E. B., & Hunt, C. (2017). Anxiety in youth with asthma: A meta-analysis. *Pediatric Pulmonology, 52*(9), 1121–1129. https://doi.org/10.1002/ppul.23689

Eccleston, C., Fisher, E., Law, E., Bartlett, J., & Palermo, T. M. (2015). Psychological interventions for parents of children and adolescents with chronic illness. *Cochrane Database of Systematic Review* (4): Art. No. CD009660, 142 p. https://doi.org/10.1002/14651858.CD009660.pub3

Ferro, M. A., & Boyle, M. H. (2015). The impact of chronic physical illness, maternal depressive symptoms, family functioning, and self-esteem on symptoms of anxiety and depression in children. *Journal of Abnormal Child Psychology, 43*, 177–187. https://doi.org/10.1007/s10802-014-9893-6

Fidler, A., Lawless, C., LaFave, E., Netz, M., McConville, A., Turner, E., & Fedele, D. (2019). Anxiety among adolescent with asthma: Relationships with asthma control and sleep quality. *Clinical Practice in Pediatric Psychology, 7*(2), 151–156. https://doi.org/10.1037/cpp0000267

Fisher, E., Heathcote, L. C., Eccleston, C., Simons, L. E., & Palermo, T. M. (2018). Assessment of pain anxiety, pain catastrophizing, and fear of pain in children and adolescents with chronic pain: A systematic review and meta-analysis. *Journal of Pediatric Psychology, 43*(3), 314–325. https://doi.org/10.1093/jpepsy/jsx103

Kendall, P. C., Settipani, C. A., & Cummings, C. M. (2012). No need to worry: The promising future of child anxiety research. *Journal of Clinical Child and Adolescent Psychology, 41*, 103–115. https://doi.org/10.1080/15374416.2012.632352

Knight, A., Weiss, P., Morales, K., Gerdes, M., Rearson, M., Vickery, M., & Keren, R. (2015). Identifying differences in risk factors for depression and anxiety in pediatric chronic disease: A matched cross-sectional study of youth with Lupus/Mixed Connective Tissue Disease and their peers with diabetes. *Journal of Pediatrics, 167*(6), 1397–1403.e1. https://doi.org/10.1016/j.jpeds.2015.07.048

Koller, D., & Goldman, R. D. (2012). Distraction techniques for children undergoing procedures: A critical review of pediatric research. *Journal of Pediatric Nursing, 27*, 652–681. https://doi.org/10.1016/j.pedn.2011.08.001

Li, W. H. C., Chung, J. O. K., Ho, K. Y., & Kwok, B. M. C. (2016). Play interventions to reduce anxiety and negative emotions in hospitalized children. *BMC Pediatrics, 16*, 36–45. https://doi.org/10.1186/s12887-016-0570-5

McCarthy, A. M., & Kleiber, C. (2006). A conceptual model of factors influencing children's responses to a painful procedure when parents are distraction coaches. *Journal of Pediatric Nursing, 21*, 88–98. https://doi.org/10.1016/j.pedn.2005.06.007

Morawska, A., Calam, R., & Fraser, J. (2015). Parenting interventions for childhood chronic illness: A review and recommendations for intervention design and delivery. *Journal of Child Health Care, 19*(1), 5–17. https://doi.org/10.1177/1367493513496664

Mullins, L. L., Molzon, E. S., Suorsa, K. I., Tackett, A. P., Pai, A. L. H., & Chaney, J. M. (2015). Models of resilience: Developing psychosocial interventions for parents of children with chronic health conditions. *Family Relations, 64*, 176–189. https://doi.org/10.1111/fare.12104

Nabors, L., & Elkins, J. (2017). *Coping positively with my worries manual for kids: Getting off the worry racetrack!* Cincinnati, OH: University of Cincinnati.

Nabors, L., Liddle, M., Graves, M. L., Kamphaus, A., & Elkins, J. (2019). A family affair: Supporting children with chronic illnesses. *Child: Care, Health and Development, 45*, 227–233. https://doi.org/10.1111/cch.12635

Nabors, L., Odar Stough, C., Combs, A., & Elkins, J. (2019). Implementing the *coping positively with my worries manual*: A pilot study. *Journal of Child and Family Studies, 28*(10), 2708–2717. https://doi.org/10.1007/s10826-019-01451-3

Norman, K. R., Silverman, W. K., & Lebowitz, E. R. (2015). Family accommodation of child and adolescent anxiety: Mannerisms, assessment, and treatment. *Journal of Child and Adolescent Psychiatric Nursing, 28*(3), 131–140. https://doi.org/10.1111/jcap.12116

Pao, M., & Bosk, A. (2011). Anxiety in medically ill children and adolescents. *Depression and Anxiety, 28*, 40–49. https://doi.org/10.1002/da.20727

Patel, A., Schieble, T., Davidson, M., Tran, M. C. J., Schoenberg, C., Delphin, E., & Bennett, H. (2006). Distraction with a hand-held video game reduces pediatric preoperative anxiety. *Pediatric Anesthesia, 16*, 1019–1027. https://doi.org/10.1111/j.1460-9592.2006.01914.x

Peterson, L., & Shigetomi, C. (1981). The use of coping techniques to minimize anxiety in hospitalized children. *Behavior Therapy, 12*(1), 1–14. https://doi.org/10.1016/S0005-7894(81)80102-5

Pinquart, M., & Shen, Y. (2011). Anxiety in children and adolescents with chronic physical illnesses: A meta-analysis. *Acta Paediatrica, 100*, 1069–1076. https://doi.org/10.1111/j.1651-2227.2011.02223.x

Quittner, A. L., Abbott, J., Georgiopoulos, A. M., Goldbeck, L., Smith, B., Hempstead, S. E., … the International Committee on Mental Health. (2016). International Committee on Mental Health in Cystic Fibrosis: Cystic Fibrosis Foundation and European Cystic Fibrosis Society consensus statements for screening and treating depression and anxiety. *Thorax, 71*, 26–34. https://doi.org/10.1136/thoraxjnl-2015-207488

Reigada, L. C., Benkov, K. J., Bruzzese, J.-M., Hoogendoorn, C., Szigeth, E., Briggie, A., … Warner, C. M. (2013). Integrating illness concerns into cognitive behavioral therapy of children and adolescents with inflammatory bowel disease and co-occurring anxiety. *Journal for Specialists in Pediatric Nursing, 18*, 133–143. https://doi.org/10.1111/jspn.12019

Stapersma, L., van den Brink, G., van der Ende, J., Szigethy, E. M., Beukers, R., Korpershoek, T. A., … Utens, E. M. W. J. (2018). Effectiveness of disease-specific cognitive behavioral therapy on anxiety, depression, and quality of life in youth with inflammatory bowel disease: A randomized controlled trial. *Journal of Pediatric Psychology, 43*(9), 967–980. https://doi.org/10.1093/jpepsy/jsy029

Stein, R. E. K., & Jessop, D. J. (1982). A noncategorical approach to chronic childhood illness. *Public Health Reports, 97*, 354–362.

Uman, L. S., Chambers, C. T., McGrath, P. J., & Kisely, S. (2008). A systematic review of randomized controlled trials examining psychological interventions for needle-related procedural pain and distress in children and adolescents: An abbreviated Cochrane review. *Journal of Pediatric Psychology, 33*, 842–854. https://doi.org/10.1093/jpepsy/jsn031

Chapter 7
Attention-Deficit Hyperactivity Disorder and Anxiety in Children

Introduction

Cuffe et al. (2015) assessed comorbid diagnoses for children with Attention-Deficit Hyperactivity Disorder (ADHD) in Oklahoma and South Carolina as part of an epidemiological study, designed to identify ADHD in elementary school-age children. There were over 200 children with ADHD in their sample. They reported that 18% of the sample had an anxiety or a mood disorder. The most common anxiety disorder was separation anxiety (about 10%) followed by social phobia (about 7%) and Generalized Anxiety Disorder (GAD, about 6%). Although children with ADHD and externalizing problems were at greater risk for difficulty in relationships and with the legal system, their findings did indicate risk for children with ADHD and anxiety:

> Children with ADHD combined with an Anxiety/Mood Disorder had the largest odds ratio for poor academic performance, but a wide confidence interval as a result of a small sample size warrants caution when interpreting this estimate (Cuffe et al., 2015, p. 5).

Tsang et al. (2015) reported that children (average age of 11 years) who had ADHD + Anxiety were more likely to experience greater severity of their ADHD symptoms. Tsang et al. (2015) found that children with the combined subtype were most likely to experience anxiety. The most common comorbid anxiety disorders in their sample included GAD and Social Anxiety Disorder. They echoed the idea that children with ADHD + anxiety may have lower educational attainment, and in adulthood these individuals may have more difficulties with occupational attainment.

Michelini, Eley, Gregory, and McAdams (2015) assessed the overlap between anxiety and ADHD in adolescence. Michelini et al. (2015) pointed out that it is valuable to consider the heterogeneity of psychiatric conditions in children. Similar to Cuffe et al. (2015), Michelini et al. (2015) reported that separation anxiety, social phobia, and GAD co-occurred with ADHD in their sample. Youth in their sample were between 12 and 19 years of age. They discovered some youth displayed

L. Nabors, *Anxiety Management in Children with Mental and Physical Health Problems*, Springer Series on Child and Family Studies,
https://doi.org/10.1007/978-3-030-35606-4_7

obsessive-compulsive symptoms. Like Cuffe et al. (2015), these authors reported a wide range in scores for anxiety symptoms. Michelini et al. (2015) reviewed genetic results, and correlations among monozygotic twins were higher than correlations among dizygotic twins. This might suggest a genetic influence. On the other hand, non-shared environmental factors were associated with symptoms. Michelini et al. (2015) called for longitudinal studies to better untangle environmental and genetic influences and determine what factors were acting on anxiety and ADHD.

Prevalence

About 9% of children aged 8–15 who reside in the USA may have ADHD (Merikangas et al., 2010). It is estimated that approximately 25% of children with ADHD present with a mood disorder, typically anxiety or depression (Cuffe et al., 2015; Reid, Graziano, McNamara, Paneto, & Geffken, 2015; Sciberras et al., 2015). Jarrett, Wolff, Davis, Cowart, and Ollendick (2012) stated that about 25% of children with ADHD experience anxiety and that this comorbidity can increase to 30–40% of youth with ADHD in the clinical population. Internalizing disorders, such as anxiety, may co-occur with ADHD in females more often than males. Specifically, in research following outcomes for children who participated in the Multimodal Treatment Study for Children with ADHD (MTA), Hinshaw, Arnold, and the MTA Cooperative Group (2015) reported ADHD was related to internalizing disorders, especially among females.

Does Comorbid Anxiety Result in Additional Deficits in Functioning?

In a pilot study, Reid et al. (2015) found that children and adolescents (6–17 years; $n = 59$) with ADHD and an anxiety disorder had fairly similar functioning to youth who were diagnosed solely with ADHD on a variety of measures. On the other hand, youth with mood disorders had more deficits in functioning than those with ADHD and anxiety or only with ADHD. Reid et al. (2015) raised the question of whether there should be an additional subtype of ADHD, specifically for ADHD and comorbid mood disorders. They thought understanding the symptoms a child or adolescent was presenting with was important, because then a therapist could take a modular approach to help the child in addressing symptoms of concern. A modular approach guides the clinician as to what interventions to try to use to ameliorate symptoms (Weisz et al., 2012). Assessing which symptoms cause the most suffering or impairment, may guide clinicians as to what to address first in treatment. Reid et al. (2015) suggested addressing ADHD symptoms may be a priority. This is an interesting idea, which bears further research.

Jarrett et al. (2012) examined performance on neurocognitive tasks for children with ADHD, children with ADHD + anxiety, and children with only anxiety. The average age of participants was 9 years (range 6–17 years). Sixty-two percent were male, and there were 39 in the ADHD only group, 30 in the ADHD + anxiety group, and 61 children in the anxiety only group. Youth in the ADHD groups showed higher variability in their scores on continuous performance tasks compared to children with only anxiety. Children with ADHD + anxiety exhibited greater deficits in working memory than children with ADHD only. Jarrett et al. (2012) speculated that higher levels of anxiety could be detrimental in that it could interfere with working memory by overloading an individual's cognitive resources.

Deficits in working memory can include difficulties with short-term memory and executive functions. Rumination or worry about events, which accompanies anxiety, may further impair working memory. Consequently, at school, teachers should write down homework assignments and use cues and reminders to assist children in focusing on classroom work. One shortcoming of their study was that their sample included mostly Caucasian youth. Characteristics of children of color who have comorbid ADHD and anxiety need to be examined. Another problem with this study was that subtypes of ADHD were not assessed. Finally, some of the children in their sample also had Oppositional Defiant Disorder (ODD), which may have exacerbated symptoms.

High-Risk Behaviors and Emotional Reactivity

Youth with ADHD may engage in risky behaviors (Humphreys & Lee, 2011). Surprisingly, worries or feelings of anxiety may be related to engaging in risky behaviors. It may be the case that engaging in a risky behavior distracts a child from feeling worries (Cooper, Agocha, & Sheldon, 2000). Another explanation may be that engaging in risky behaviors fits with the notion of being high in "sensation seeking" and having difficulty with emotion regulation, which may occur during adolescence. If this does occur, then adolescents with ADHD and anxiety may engage in more risky behaviors, especially if they are male (Arbel, Perrone, & Margolin, 2018). Engaging in risky behaviors may exacerbate worries, and alternating cycles of worry leading to risky behaviors and vice versa may develop (Arbel et al., 2018). Seeking support from others, such as counselors and mentors, may buffer adolescents in terms of reducing risk and worry. Positive interactions with friends and family members "... appear to contain some of the reverberating effects between worries and risky behaviors" (Arbel et al., 2018, p. 909). Texting or talking about "daily concerns" (Arbel et al., 2018, p. 909) was perceived as supportive by teenagers. There can be times when the support of peers can backfire, however. This may occur when teenagers perceive the interaction with a peer as negative (making them feel badly for reaching out for support). If reaching for support turns negative, it can spur worries and fuel the worry–risk behavior cycle.

Many children and adolescents with ADHD face difficulties with emotion regulation, and those with relatively lower abilities in this area may have higher levels of impairment in their relationships and functioning (Anastopoulos et al., 2011). Difficulty with emotion regulation may lie at the heart of some "transdiagnostic" interventions for youth with ADHD and anxiety. Schneider, Arch, and Landy (2018) examined how emotion regulation is related to anxiety. Schneider et al. (2018) referred to Gross and Thompson's (2007) definition of emotion regulation as, "… involving a set of processes through which emotions are modified, changed or managed" (Schneider et al., 2018, p. 978). These authors discussed the importance of helping children and adolescents become aware of their emotions and learn the ability to "watch" or process emotions as they occur without reacting or acting. Children and adolescents with attentional problems and anxiety may benefit from becoming more aware of the fact that emotions are dictating their reactions. If they can learn to watch and evaluate their emotions before acting or reacting, they have the potential to achieve better interpersonal outcomes. Intervention techniques designed to help youth understand and regulate their emotions will help reduce social and interaction difficulties related to ADHD and anxiety.

Teaching children to become mindful of the present, the emotions they feel, and the value of using problem-solving before reacting can have a positive impact on avoidance associated with anxiety and impulsive responses. Studying one's emotions can reduce emotional lability (Schneider et al., 2018). Engaging in goal-directed behavior as well as considering what one wants to achieve before reacting emotionally can help children and adolescents control reactive and dysregulated behavioral responses (Schneider et al., 2018). Committed action—where children and adolescents focus on what they want their behaviors to be, while learning techniques to stop and reset negative emotional reactions—may be instrumental in helping them act and think themselves into new behaviors (Blackledge & Hayes, 2001). Children and adolescents also can engage in opposite reaction. Thus, rather than becoming angry or upset, they can practice engaging in the opposite reaction, which enables them to exhibit a positive behavior. Then, hopefully, the child or the adolescent will receive positive reinforcement or praise after this positive reaction, which encourages further positive behaviors (Blackledge & Hayes, 2001; Schneider et al., 2018).

Treatment

Hinshaw et al. (2015) presented interesting information about how children with ADHD and anxiety responded to medication and counseling (i.e., behavioral therapy). They found that youth with ADHD and a comorbid anxiety disorder often responded positively to medication, medication + behavioral therapy, and behavioral therapy equally. If the child had anxiety and ADHD, then parents and health professionals should consider behavioral therapy as a frontline treatment. Behavioral therapy can assist the child with building positive habits (e.g., positive ways of responding and positive behaviors) and can assist the parent(s) and child in building social skills and positive behavioral skills (Hinshaw et al., 2015). Hinshaw et al. (2015) concluded that behavioral therapy helped children with ADHD function better socially, both at home and in the classroom. They stated that behavioral therapy has benefits after treatment ends; but, the impact of medication ends when it no longer is in the child's system. If a child has ADHD, it is valuable to add parent training to treatment, and to work with parents to reduce ineffective and negative parenting practices. They proposed that combined behavioral therapy and medication management should be considered a frontline treatment for children with ADHD and anxiety. They believed parental discipline (e.g., positive instructions and structure) was key to improving behaviors (for children with ADHD—irrespective of whether they presented with anxiety). It is noteworthy that they did not provide guidance as to what treatment is best for which specific type of anxiety disorder.

In a pilot study, Sciberras et al. (2015) conducted a randomized controlled trial to determine the effectiveness of the "Cool Kids Program" for children with ADHD and anxiety. Participants were children aged 8–12 with ADHD, who were recruited from an ADHD clinic. There were five boys who participated in treatment and six boys in a treatment as usual group. Those children in the treatment group participated in the Cool Kids Program, which was developed by Rapee et al. (2013). Sciberras et al. (2015) modified this program to allow more breaks between activities, added an activity schedule, and stressed repetition of key ideas. During programming they reinforced on task behaviors. A key component of Rapee et al.'s (2013) Cool Kids Program was psychoeducation for parents and children to reduce avoidance and increase children's involvement in activities and with peers. In vivo exposure is used to expose children to anxiety-provoking situations. Children learn problem-solving skills and ideas for improving social interactions. Moreover, children learn to be worry detectives to understand situations in which they worry and determine whether excessive fears are necessary. Parents learn the aforementioned ideas to help their child manage his or her anxiety (Rapee et al., 2013). At the end of the program, Sciberras et al. (2015) reported that all of the children in the treatment as usual group still had their anxiety diagnosis, while three of the children in the modified Cool Kids Program were anxiety free. Children in the treatment group reported improved quality of life and parents and teachers reported improved child functioning. Sciberras et al. (2015) concluded that if left untreated, anxiety may increase symptoms of ADHD and that anxiety may not remit without treatment.

It has been my experience that children with anxiety and ADHD may face low self-esteem related to their impulsive behaviors. Their anxiety may add to feelings of poor self-esteem if the child has an "I can't do it" attitude and gets too down on himself or herself. Other children may work hard to hold their behavior "together" during the school day. When returning home, they may become very "hyper" as they "let off steam." Others may face "rebound" when they come home, as their ADHD medications are "wearing off"/leaving their systems. Medication leaving the child's system or "wearing off" may exacerbate feelings of agitation and "moodiness," which, in turn, can contribute to feelings of worry. Further, if children or adolescents are tired and agitated, because their medication is no longer working, they may experience heightened anxiety. This may increase behavioral refusal—and children/adolescents may refuse to do chores and/or homework. This has the potential to become a cycle, with ever-increasing negative impact that can impede abilities to finish homework. If a child with ADHD + anxiety faces difficulty with working memory, perhaps because anxiety drains or overtasks cognitive resources (Jarrett et al., 2012), then a child may have further difficulty concentrating on school work and with recalling or writing down homework. For these children, training to improve organizational skills and requiring a teacher check planners or homework lists, to ensure that all homework is recorded, can be helpful.

Family-Oriented Cognitive Behavior Therapy

Maric, van Steensel, and Bögels (2015) examined the effectiveness of a child cognitive-behavioral therapy (CBT) intervention versus a family CBT intervention for children with anxiety and ADHD. Participants for their study were part of a larger research study to treat anxiety in children using a CBT protocol (e.g., Bodden et al., 2008). Forty-nine children with ADHD and anxiety participated in child CBT and 37 children with ADHD and anxiety participated in family CBT. Children ranged in age from 8 to 18 years. For the child-based CBT condition, treatment was 13 sessions using a treatment manual. Sessions covered education about anxiety, exposure, cognitive restructuring, and ideas for preventing relapse of symptoms related to anxiety. In terms of exposure and cognitive restructuring, Maric et al. (2015) mentioned that a goal was to reduce anxiety through using a fear hierarchy, allowing for graded exposure to feared stimuli/events and opportunities to change dysfunctional thinking. Children could receive rewards for moving through their fear hierarchy. Parents were involved in learning about their child's fear hierarchy and parents participated in educational sessions to learn about anxiety.

Family-based CBT sessions (Maric et al., 2015) included sessions for children and parents that involved education about anxiety, ideas for reducing cognitive thinking errors, and ideas for reducing fears through graded exposures. In additional parenting sessions, parents learned to identify and cope with their own dysfunctional beliefs and to identify and resolve problems in family interactions and communications. Problem-solving was added to help improve dysfunctional family interactions and communication styles. During family-based CBT, five more parent sessions were held and there were two parent and child sessions. There were three sessions for children. Three sessions involved the entire family—including siblings. Maric et al. (2015) concluded that the children with ADHD plus anxiety did benefit from family sessions, perhaps because the family training allowed clinicians to address negative parenting strategies and family patterns that were not helpful for children with ADHD. Parents could help their children to focus and pay attention; therefore, the children were better able to learn anxiety management strategies.

Maric et al. (2015) reported that younger children responded better to treatment compared to older youth. This may be due to the large role of contingency management in their program—with the anxiety hierarchy and rewards. It may be more difficult for parents to help with this type of intervention for older children and teenagers. It is noteworthy that the sample sizes were small when age was considered, and further study is needed. For adolescents and teenagers, more self-directed anxiety management strategies, which allow the child to use relaxation and distraction to reset physiologically, and cognitive strategies to power through anxiety situations, may be helpful interventions. It is remarkable that the children in the groups for Maric et al.'s (2015) study did not have significant levels of ADHD symptomology. Accordingly, use of these types of treatments needs to be replicated in samples where children and adolescents are exhibiting clinically elevated levels of ADHD symptoms.

Jarrett and Ollendick (2012) developed a combined treatment approach involving parent management training and family cognitive behavioral training. The parent training (to work with ADHD) involved lessons on helping children with skills to improve executive functioning, such as homework completion, as well as teaching parents about reinforcement and behavior management techniques, like response costs for misbehavior. These authors added anxiety management skills training for parents. The use of response costs was made optional, which is good because some parents might not wish to use this technique. Time spent positively attending to the child was also part of their program. They adapted treatments from Barkley's (1997) *Defiant Child* as well as techniques from Rapee, Wignall, Hudson, and Schniering's (2000) Cool Kid's Program, which has family-based treatment at the heart of treatment of children's anxiety (Rapee et al., 2000). Sessions from Rapee et al.'s (2000) program were shortened with breaks and rewards for children with ADHD. Jarrett and Ollendick (2012) had eight children and their parents enrolled in the pilot study. Four of the children were boys. Single case designs with multiple baselines were used to evaluate implementation of the intervention. Seven of the eight families completed the 10-week treatment. Results showed gains in management of anxiety symptoms and some gains in management of ADHD symptoms (Jarrett & Ollendick, 2012). The gains in managing anxiety were still positive at a 6-month follow-up. Their sample size was small and treatments were not delivered sequentially; hence, more research is needed.

Mindfulness as "Added Value" to Treatment Approaches

Mindfulness interventions may add value to existing treatment protocols for children with ADHD and anxiety (e.g., van der Oord, Bögels, & Peijenenburg, 2012). Parents and children receive sensory training, participate in yoga, and learn to meditate and be mindful in their actions (see van der Oord et al. (2012) for a description of a possible intervention package for small groups of children and parents). Moreover, Bögels and her colleagues provide a detailed description of "mindful" parenting, based on using meditation to center the self and to learn to review situations in a thoughtful, solution-oriented manner (Bögels, Lehtonen, & Restifo,

2010). Being more mindful and relaxed may address both symptoms of anxiety and ADHD. Participating in these types of interventions may reduce parental reactivity and withdrawal from the child. It may relieve parent stress as well, if parents are practicing mindfulness techniques along with their children. When parents learn to be mindful, it may allow them to take a break and reset mentally and physiologically when coping with challenging child behaviors. After they have examined their stress and perhaps relaxed, they may be recharged to implement interventions.

When parents are mindful, then they may be more likely to engage with their child, while supporting the child by granting him or her autonomy. The positive support can be empowering for children, leading to improved "uptake" of new behaviors, which may lead to improved behavioral outcomes. When the parent is not avoiding the child and actively engaged with him or her, there can be reduced anxiety for the child and the parent. Having parents available to guide and support the child's behaviors may improve progress for children with ADHD and anxiety, by decreasing child anxiety and allowing parents to reinforce positive behaviors. Externalizing behaviors could be reduced if the child is calmer and a parent is "present" to model and teach the child how to control and cope with emotional reactivity. The parent becomes a positive role model of "regulated" behaviors and positive problem-solving for the child, which could be positive in changing child behavior and improving emotion regulation.

Manassis et al. (2014) recommended parent involvement in therapy, because it may facilitate "... generalization of skills in 'real-world' settings." (p. 1164). Parents can have an instrumental role in reinforcing positive behaviors for children with ADHD and they can play a critical role in rewarding children for confronting and moving through anxiety-provoking events (e.g., using graded exposure). I use reinforcement charts for preschool-age and elementary school-age children. These charts typically have one goal for preschool children and two to three goals for elementary schoolers. There are short-term rewards, like a piece of candy provided when a parent observes a positive or prosocial behavior, such as completing a task per parent instructions (goal for ADHD) or not erasing work on a homework paper (goal for anxiety). If a child has several successes (e.g., several checks on a chart for a goal) then he or she can earn a higher-level reward, like a small toy or playing a game with a parent. The parent decides on rewards, learns about prompting desired behaviors, and selects the rewards (sometimes children help in selecting rewards as well). This involves parent training, which can occur during the session with the child and/or during individual sessions. This transfer of control to the parent can "stretch" the impact of treatment promoting skill development and generalization of training, resulting in long-term positive behavioral outcomes (Manassis et al., 2014).

Case Studies

There are two cases, one with an adolescent (shorter in length) and then a case with a younger child.

Case One The first case focuses on, Jake, who is a 14-year-old freshman, having difficulty with anxiety and some sadness due to a bullying episode. He has a history of ADHD. Recently, he was hospitalized for being depressed and anxious. After a short stay, he was released to be followed by a psychiatrist, who prescribed antidepressants and to participate in counseling to work on symptoms of anxiety as well as his feelings of sadness. In terms of treating anxiety, Jake and his therapist worked on stopping to evaluate his thoughts, while stepping back, relaxing, and realizing his strong emotions, without letting them determine his behavior. Learning to be mindful, to stop, relax, and think about his emotions was a central component of treatment. Jake tended to be very reactive and reported, "I don't have any thoughts. I just act." The therapist continued to work with Jake to identify emotions, his self-talk, and to stop and reflect before acting. During sessions, Jake "replayed" situations that he had experienced at school and with peers. He learned to identify his feelings and began to problem-solve, regarding the antecedents to his feelings, his feelings, automatic behaviors, and then "thinking" or problem-solving to reflect on how his reactions/behaviors could foster positive interactions.

Jake mentioned he was often "down" on himself. He tended to talk negatively to himself and see others' actions as having negative outcomes for him. He had a hostile bias, thinking that peers were "out for themselves" and wanted to hurt others to get ahead. This hostile attribution bias has been discussed by many researchers (e.g., de Castro, Veerman, Koops, Bosch, & Monshouwer, 2002). Jake tended to behave aggressively or experience anxiety related to this way of thinking. Furthermore, feelings of worry could also be translated to aggression, because being aggressive was more "normal for a guy" than being worried, in Jake's opinion.

The therapist used role play, with "stop and think" checks, to teach Jake to review situations in order to learn that his peers might not have hostile intentions in social exchanges. Moreover, Jake implemented a thought record—to begin to write his thoughts in a journal. After identifying his thoughts, he recorded his feelings in what became his "thoughts and feelings notes." He learned he had many feelings and one of them was extreme anxiety about others judging him negatively and extreme worry over impulsivity related to his ADHD. In a joint session, the therapist and Jake's mother worked with him to realize that his feelings did not need to be translated into negative reactions when he was very upset. They role-played different situations with Jake, and he began to identify his negative feelings, negative self-talk, and impulsive behaviors that were ineffective with peers and resulted in negative consequences for him (such as impulsive use of Instagram to release negative feelings about friends). Jake learned to stop, relax, take a break from the cellular telephone and "instant communication," and think through his responses to others. After a few weeks of practice, he and his mother reported more positive responses to others and more positive texts and posts. Jake reported reduced anxiety. He enjoyed relaxation—which he accomplished through slow breathing and positive imagery of him surfing waves (his favorite activity). Subsequent to reducing impulsivity and decreasing anxiety over social interactions, Jake reported improved self-esteem and improved interpersonal relationships.

Case Two Susie was a 6-year-old girl whose mother stated she had been diagnosed with ADHD. She was taking a small dose of a stimulant medication to treat her ADHD. Unfortunately, Susie was still having "meltdowns" about her homework in the afternoons. She would refuse to complete her work if she did not understand instructions or made even one mistake on a multiproblem homework assignment. Her mother described Susie as being a perfectionist, who could not tolerate any mistake on her work or who felt embarrassed if she could not understand how to do her homework. Susie's mother reported that she had the same "issues" as Susie when she was a child. Her teacher helped her cope by giving her additional work to complete. Upon further questioning, Susie's mother admitted she had to have her art work completed perfectly or she would rip up the paper or destroy the art project and begin it again.

The therapist contacted Susie's teacher, because Susie was having some difficulty with being out of her seat and talking to others when she and her classmates needed to be working quietly on assignments. They discussed use of a reward chart with intermediate rewards for good daily behavior (e.g., not talking to others, following instructions, and completing her seat work). Susie's teacher would "catch her on task" and she would receive a check on her goal chart for "working on her assignment" or "not talking" to others when it was quiet work time (immediate reinforcers). Moreover, a school-home note was implemented so that Susie's teacher could inform her parents about her daily behavioral progress. In terms of intermediate rewards, if Susie had five checks on her goal chart she could earn a small prize, such as an eraser from the prize box in the classroom.

If she had three good days per week, then her parents would purchase a small toy for her and she earned a prize from the teacher's prize box (high-level reward). Susie's parents received update information on her progress on the goal sheet for her classroom through a school-home note. Her teacher instructed the teacher's assistant on the program. The therapist taught both the teacher and teacher's assistant to check and ensure that Susie was doing her work and provide gentle reminders to remain on task. The therapist worked with the teacher, reviewing the use of cues, such as, "Susie, be on your 'A' game," as a cue for Susie to work on her classroom assignments. The therapist worked with Susie, using role play, so she understood the cue was meant to help her remember to focus on her classroom work. The therapist also introduced the reward chart to Susie and explained how the teacher would implement the chart.

The therapist worked with Susie's teacher to ensure that she wrote down homework for Susie. Susie had a new "finish" folder where she placed her school work after it was completed. She used this folder at school and at home. The therapist taught Susie and her mother how to organize Susie's backpack, how to use her finished folder for keeping track of her completed homework, and how to develop a homework checklist for completing each night's assigned tasks. The therapist explained treatment to the teacher on subsequent telephone contacts. Moreover, Susie's mother "timed" her homework so that Susie could work for 15 min and then take a 5-min movement break. Susie completed her homework immediately after having snack. When her homework was completed, then she could go outside and play.

Susie's mother and father used a similar reward chart at home. Their chart was very similar to the one at school; but, it included a "go to bed by the third request" goal. Susie received short-term (small piece of candy for two checks on her chart), intermediate (very small toy for four to five checks), and weekly rewards (e.g., a trip to the store for a small toy for ten to twelve checks). Her goals were to listen to instructions and try to carry them out, do her homework, and go to bed on time each evening. It is valuable to use rewards for children with ADHD and to remember that some children with ADHD may be less sensitive to negative feedback or consequences (e.g., Humphreys & Lee, 2011).

Unfortunately, after a month, Susie still could not complete her homework. She was not earning any rewards for completion of homework. The therapist wondered if her medication was still working at home or if she was "rebounding" from the medication. A referral was made to Susie's pediatrician for a medication evaluation. Her pediatrician prescribed a small dose of Ritalin in the afternoons. After this, Susie was able to be successful in completing her homework. She was able to listen to instructions and was going to bed—typically by the second or third reminder from her parents. This was a big improvement. As Susie's behavior improved, her tantrums and negative behaviors decreased. She was less anxious and no longer bit her fingernails, which her parents reported were signs of her being worried at the initiation of treatment.

Susie's mother had become stressed with the homework struggles and was feeling somewhat disconnected from her daughter. The therapist worked with Susie's mother to practice meditation. After her mother became proficient with meditation, she tried using a quick 1-min meditation cue to focus herself before working with Susie on her homework. She encouraged Susie to decrease her anxiety over making her homework "perfect." Susie's mother reported that the meditation reduced her own anxiety, which was often high after a hard day at work. It helped her focus on "just being a mother and working with my child."

A relaxation approach was used to help Susie stop worrying about her homework papers being perfect. The therapist instructed Susie's mother about how to teach Susie to use breathing to relax when she felt upset about stray marks on her paper or when she did not immediately understand her homework. Susie would take six deep breaths and then use her super-cat superhero to help her think about "I can try" statements. This was written on an index card ("I can try"), with Susie's picture of her super-hero cat named "Addy the Mighty." The therapist role-played with Susie—teaching her to use breathing and her superhero "cue card." Her mother observed this session. Susie's mother relayed the relaxation strategy to Susie's teacher and the therapist followed up with a telephone call to review the relaxation exercise. She requested the teacher, like her mother, encourage Susie to turn in her work even if it was not perfect. The therapist requested that both Susie's mother and her teacher not allow her to have a new piece of paper or a new worksheet every time she noticed a stray mark on the page. It was difficult for Susie, but after having to turn in her homework sheets "as they were" (with stray marks) a few times, she learned to power through (using breathing and positive self-talk), finishing her work, even if there was an erased mark or stray mark on her homework sheet. Communication with the teacher allowed her to use the "can do" statements and an "Addy Card" while Susie was working on classroom assignments.

The therapist also talked with Susie about her worries. They talked about other feelings that were behind the worries, such as not liking to do homework. They discussed her worries about thinking she would not do well and get something wrong when she was completing her homework. When Susie, her mother, and the therapist talked about "timing" her homework completion, they talked about brief checks of homework by Susie's mother during her movement time. Susie's mother would check the work during these breaks. After the movement break had ended, her mother would answer any questions and provide feedback on the homework. Susie responded well to this. During the first week of this intervention, Susie got a reward if she had a stray mark on her paper and had not erased it or torn up her paper. If she got a problem wrong, then she and her mother practiced saying, "It's OK, I'm learning." Her mother and teacher would tell Susie, "If you get a problem wrong, then you can always learn an answer that will work." She practiced slow breathing (taking five or six slow breaths) if she needed to remain calm. This breathing and positive practice reduced Susie's anxiety, and she began completing her homework.

Susie learned to identify her feelings and use her "words" to express how she was feeling. Increasing her feelings vocabulary and improving her self-expression reduced tantrums at home. Role play with dolls during the session provided Susie with a non-threatening way to learn about the impact of her tantrums on others and learn new ways to respond. As she learned to use her words, her mother was simultaneously reporting that Susie seemed less worried. Nail biting was decreasing. During this time, Susie learned to use the steps to the second floor of her home as her calm-down spot, where she went to breathe and practice calming down a pretend "Addy Cat" who she held in her arms or who sat on her lap. Susie really liked cats, and calming her pretend cat while breathing helped her take a break when she felt upset. Using her words became a new way of communicating with her parents. During this process it became apparent that Susie became worried when she was impulsive and not able to pay attention, because she wanted to please her parents. Armed with this new understanding, her parents were able to slow down and work to provide clear instructions and transition warnings (warnings when Susie would have to switch to a new activity). This further reduced Susie's worry and reactivity over the course of the day.

The description of Susie and her response was very positive. It is essential to remember that young children with ADHD and/or oppositional behaviors may be less cooperative, more impulsive, and less persistent than children with anxiety (Melegari et al., 2015). When these conditions co-occur, therapists and parents should adjust interventions and expectations. Interventions should be shorter, with frequent rewards to encourage a "can do" attitude. Reward charts should focus on providing rewards, rather than taking away points for misbehavior. If points are taken away, the child can feel discouraged and worry can ensue, causing them to "give up" and stop trying to follow goals on the reward chart. Parents should try to make sure that they are looking at the child and providing short sentences when giving instructions. Teaching strategies, like breathing and self-calming strategies, can help improve emotion regulation, which is a hallmark of positive functioning for young children (Melegari et al., 2015).

Conclusions

Research has shown that treatments for ADHD and anxiety can be successful for children with both disorders (e.g., Jarrett & Ollendick, 2012). Comorbid anxiety can exacerbate symptoms, if a child is worrying because he or she is having difficulty following instructions and completing tasks. Positive support and frequent, concrete rewards can help the child gain self-confidence and persist in working to improve his or her behaviors. Maric et al. (2015) reported that young children responded relatively better than adolescents to use of a graded hierarchy to treat anxiety symptoms. Hinshaw et al. (2015) proposed that parental involvement and positive discipline could make a difference in children's developmental trajectories. Parents may have ADHD or anxiety; therefore, a mindful approach may help them to react mindfully and focus on helping their child achieve positive outcomes in terms of improved behaviors and reduced anxiety at home. The case studies focused on reviewing techniques to work with children, parents, and teachers. Reward charts, with immediate and longer-term rewards, help with goal attainment. Breathing and relaxation may help with anxiety and help the child or adolescent self-monitor his or her emotional state, thereby helping with impulsive responding related to having ADHD. Future research needs to examine which strategies are "best matched" for which type ADHD (e.g., inattention or combined symptoms) and which type of anxiety (GAD, phobias, separation anxiety, etc.).

References

Anastopoulos, A. D., Smith, T. F., Garrett, M. E., Morrissey-Kane, E., Schatz, N. K., Sommer, J. L., … Ashley-Koch, A. (2011). Self-regulation of emotion, functional impairment, and comorbidity among children with AD/HD. *Journal of Attention Disorders, 15*(7), 583–592. https://doi.org/10.1177/1087054710370567

Arbel, R., Perrone, L., & Margolin, G. (2018). Adolescents' daily worries and risky behaviors: The buffering role of support seeking. *Journal of Clinical Child and Adolescent Psychology, 47*(6), 900–911. https://doi.org/10.1080/15374416.2016.1169536

Barkley, R. A. (1997). *Defiant children: A clinician's manual for parent training* (2nd ed.). New York, NY: Guilford Press.

Blackledge, J. T., & Hayes, S. C. (2001). Emotion regulation in acceptance and commitment therapy. *Journal of Clinical Psychology, 57*(2), 243–255. https://doi.org/10.1002/(ISSN)1097-4679

Bodden, D. H. M., Bögels, S. M., Nauta, M. H., De Haan, E., Ringrose, J., Appelboom, C., … Appleboom-Gerts, K. C. (2008). Child versus family cognitive-behavioral therapy in clinically anxious youth: An efficacy and partial effectiveness study. *Journal of American Academy of Child and Adolescent Psychiatry, 47*(12), 1384–1394. https://doi.org/10.1097/CHI.0b013e318189148e

Bögels, S. M., Lehtonen, A., & Restifo, K. (2010, May, Online). Mindful parenting in mental health care. *Mindfulness, 1*, 107–120. https://doi.org/10.1007/s12671-010-0014-5. downloaded August 3, 2019

Cooper, M. L., Agocha, V. B., & Sheldon, M. S. (2000). A motivational perspective on risky behaviors: The role of personality and affect regulatory processes. *Journal of Personality, 68*, 1059–1088. https://doi.org/10.1111/1467-6494.00126

Cuffe, S. P., Visser, S. N., Holbrook, J. R., Danielson, M. L., Geryk, L. L., Wolraich, M. L., & McKeown, R. E. (2015, November, Online). Attention-Deficit/Hyperactivity Disorder and psychiatric comorbidity: Functional outcomes in a school-based sample of children. *Journal of Attention Disorders*, Epub version, 10p. https://doi.org/10.1177/1087054715613437. downloaded August 3, 2019

de Castro, B. O., Veerman, J. W., Koops, W., Bosch, J. D., & Monshouwer, H. J. (2002). Hostile attribution of intent and aggressive behavior: A meta-analysis. *Child Development, 73*(3), 916–932. https://doi.org/10.1111/1467-8634.00447

Gross, J. J., & Thompson, R. A. (2007). Emotion regulation. Conceptual foundations. In J. Gross (Ed.), *Handbook of emotion regulation* (pp. 3–24). New York: NY: Guilford Press.

Hinshaw, S. P., Arnold, L. E., & the MTA Cooperative Group. (2015). ADHD, multimodal treatment and longitudinal outcome: Evidence, paradox, and challenge. *Interdisciplinary Reviews in Cognitive Science, 6*(1), 39–52. https://doi.org/10.1002/wcs.1324

Humphreys, K. L., & Lee, S. S. (2011). Risk taking and sensitivity to punishment in children with ADHD, ODD, and ADHD + ODD, and controls. *Journal of Psychopathology and Behavioral Assessment, 33*(3), 299–307. https://doi.org/10.1007/s10862-011-9237-6

Jarrett, M. A., & Ollendick, T. H. (2012). Treatment of comorbid attention-deficit/hyperactivity disorder and anxiety in children: A multiple baseline analysis. *Journal of Consulting and Clinical Psychology, 80*(2), 239–244. https://doi.org/10.1037/a0027123

Jarrett, M. A., Wolff, J. C., Davis, T. E., III, Cowart, M. J., & Ollendick, T. H. (2012, August, Online). Characteristics of children with ADHD and comorbid anxiety. *Journal of Attention Disorders*, published online, 9p. https://journals.sagepub.com/doi/abs/10.1177/1087054712452914?journalCode=jada. downloaded August 3, 2019

Manassis, K., Lee, T. C., Bennett, K., Zhao, X. Y., Mendlowitz, S., Duda, S., … Wood, J. J. (2014). Types of parental involvement in CBT with anxious youth: A preliminary meta-analysis. *Journal of Consulting and Clinical Psychology, 82*(6), 1163–1172. https://doi.org/10.1037/a0036969

Maric, M., van Steensel, F. J. A., & Bögels, S. M. (2015, March, Online). Parental involvement in CBT for anxiety-disordered youth revisited: Family CBT outperforms child CBT in the long term for children with comorbid ADHD symptoms. *Journal of Attention Disorders*, published online, 9p. https://doi.org/10.1177/1087054715573991. downloaded on August 3, 2019

Melegari, M. G., Nanni, V., Lucidi, F., Russo, P. M., Donfrancesco, R., & Cloninger, C. R. (2015). Temperament and character profiles of preschool children with ODD, ADHD, and anxiety disorders. *Comprehensive Psychiatry, 58*, 94–101. https://doi.org/10.1016/j.comppsych.2015.01.001

Merikangas, K. R., Jian-Ping, H., Brody, D., Fisher, P. W., Bourdon, K., & Koretz, D. S. (2010). Prevalence and treatment of mental disorders among US children in the 2001–2004 NHANES. *Pediatrics, 125*(1), 75–81. https://doi.org/10.1542/peds.2008-2598

Michelini, G., Eley, T. C., Gregory, A. M., & McAdams, T. A. (2015). Aetiological overlap between anxiety and attention deficit hyperactivity symptom dimensions in adolescence. *Journal of Child Psychology and Psychiatry, 56*(4), 423–431. https://doi.org/10.1111/jcpp.12318

Rapee, R. M., Lyneham, H. J., Hudson, J. L., Kangas, M., Wuthrich, V. M., & Schniering, C. A. (2013). Effect of comorbidity on treatment of anxious children and adolescents: Results from a large combined sample. *Journal of the American Academy of Child and Adolescent Psychiatry, 52*, 48–58. https://doi.org/10.1016/j/jaac.2012.10.002

Rapee, R. M., Wignall, A., Hudson, J. L., & Schniering, C. A. (2000). *Treating anxious children and adolescents: An evidence-based approach*. Oakland, CA: New Harbinger.

Reid, A., Graziano, P., McNamara, J., Paneto, A., & Geffken, G. (2015). Functional impairment differences among youth with ADHD: The role of comorbid anxiety and mood disorders. *Journal of Nature And Science, 1*(1), e31. http://www.jnsci.org/index.php?journal=nsci&page=article&op=view&path%5B%5D=31. downloaded August 3, 2019

Schneider, R. L., Arch, J. J., & Landy, L. N. (2018). The longitudinal effect of emotion regulation strategies on anxiety levels in children and adolescents. *Journal of Clinical Child and Adolescent Psychology, 47*(6), 978–991. https://doi.org/10.1080/15374416.2016.1157757

Sciberras, E., Mulraney, M., Anderson, V., Rapee, R. M., Nicholson, J. M., Efron, D., … & Hiscock, H. (2015, May, Online). Managing anxiety in children with ADHD using cognitive-behavioral therapy: A pilot randomized controlled trial. *Journal of Attention Disorders*, published online, 7p. https://journals.sagepub.com/doi/abs/10.1177/1087054715584054?journalCode=jada. downloaded on August 3, 2019

Tsang, T. W., Kohn, M. R., Efron, D., Clarke, S. D., Clark, C. R., Lamb, C., & Williams, L. M. (2015). Anxiety in young people with ADHD: Clinical and self-report outcomes. *Journal of Attention Disorders, 19*(1), 18–26. https://doi.org/10.1177/1087054712446830

Van der Oord, S., Bögels, S. M., & Peijenenburg, D. (2012). The effectiveness of mindfulness training for children with ADHD and mindful parenting for their parents. *Journal of Child and Family Studies, 21*(1), 139–147. https://doi.org/10.1007/s10826-011-9457-0

Weisz, J. R., Chorpita, B. F., Palinkas, L. A., Schoenwalk, S. K., Miranda, J., Bearman, S. K., … Gibbons, R. D. (2012). Testing standard and modular designs for psychotherapy treating depression, anxiety and conduct problems in youth: A randomized effectiveness trial. *Archives of General Psychiatry, 69*(3), 274–282. https://doi.org/10.1001/archgenpsychiatry.2011.147

Chapter 8
Conduct Problems and Anxiety in Children

Introduction

Youth with Conduct Disorders (CD) often engage in behaviors that hurt others, which include violating the rights of others, violating social norms and rules, and violating behavioral expectations (e.g., engaging in aggressive and possibly violent behavior toward others; American Psychiatric Association (DSM-V), 2013, Blair, Leibenluft, & Pine, 2014; Kazdin, 1997). Kazdin (1997) described aggression, destruction of property, fire-setting, and stealing as potential behaviors related to CD in children and adolescents. Youth with CD may have higher levels of reactive aggression, where they react with aggression and hostility to actions by others (Euler et al., 2015). Children with CD often meet criteria for other behavior problems. One of these is Attention-Deficit Hyperactivity Disorder (Blair et al., 2014) and another is anxiety (Bubier & Drabick, 2009).

Oppositional Defiant Disorder (ODD) is discussed in tandem with CD in this chapter and both are referred to as conduct problems. These two disorders frequently co-occur (Kazdin, 1997). However, CD is separated from ODD by intensity of problems, with CD being more severe. Youth with ODD have irritable mood, disruptive and problem behaviors, are argumentative and defiant, and can be vindictive toward others (American Psychiatric Association (DSM-V), 2013). The characteristics of ODD and CD interfere with children's lives or daily functioning and can be present in the preschool years, with rates of disruptive behaviors being higher in males compared to females. Genetic predisposition or factors, such as having a difficult temperament (e.g., being unable to regulate and control one's emotions and poor frustration tolerance), may be a hallmark feature for those with conduct problems. Other features may be reduced cortisol in the brain, differences in prefrontal activity in the cortex, and lower heart rates (American Psychiatric Association (DSM-V), 2013; Tolan, Dodge, & Rutter, 2013). ODD and CD occur in about 4%

L. Nabors, *Anxiety Management in Children with Mental and Physical Health Problems*, Springer Series on Child and Family Studies,
https://doi.org/10.1007/978-3-030-35606-4_8

of children, with prevalence rates increasing in the adolescent years (American Psychiatric Association (DSM-V), 2013). The two most common forms of co-occurring anxiety are Generalized Anxiety Disorder and Social Anxiety Disorder (e.g., Bubier & Drabick, 2009). However, these may be the types of anxiety one reads about most frequently, because they are more common diagnoses for children and adolescents.

Bubier and Drabick (2009) reviewed the literature and discussed relations among anxiety and disruptive behaviors, including ADHD, ODD, and CD. They proposed the association among these mental health problems could come from anxiety resulting in disruptive behaviors. However, the most common pathway was from disruptive behaviors leading to anxiety. They suggested five possible explanations for the co-occurrence of anxiety and conduct problems. One is that there is a neurochemical underpinning and both dopamine and serotonin may be implicated in the expression of anxious and disruptive behaviors. Second, it may be that the behaviors are learned in interactions with parents, and there is a possibility that parents do not pay attention to positive behavioral interactions. Third, disruptive behaviors may be learned from others in the child's life—for instance, Bubier and Drabick (2009) pointed to the higher levels of disruptive and negative behaviors among children who grow up in neighborhoods where there are high levels of violence. Fourth, they mentioned that children with anxiety and conduct problems may process information differently (e.g., seeing others actions as hostile) such that there may be information processing deficits that underlie the co-occurrence of conduct problems and anxiety. Fifth, they mentioned children having what might be described as a "difficult" temperament are characterized by having difficulty regulating emotions.

Melegari et al. (2015) believed that temperament was critical in its relationship with conduct problems and anxiety. They assessed preschool temperament, including harm avoidance and novelty seeking, for children with ODD and anxiety. They found that preschool-age children with anxiety were relatively low in novelty seeking and higher in terms of harm avoidance. In contrast, children with ODD were likely to be characterized as harm avoidant but were high in novelty seeking. It may be that the being less likely to seek novelty and engage in risk behaviors is protective, when youth have conduct problems, like ODD and anxiety. Melegari et al. (2015) did not examine comorbid traits. Therefore, this idea is speculative and bears further investigation.

Children and adolescents with several (more than two) comorbid disorders may have poorer functioning. Blair et al. (2014) noted some overlap with Autism Spectrum Disorder (ASD), conduct problems, and anxiety. Storch et al. (2012) discussed these types of overlapping symptoms. They discovered that children with ASD who exhibited high levels of disruptive behaviors had higher levels of anxiety, and were more likely to be prescribed antipsychotic medications. Unfortunately, children with three levels of symptoms were not more likely to receive additional treatment (Storch et al., 2012). Those youth with more severe symptoms may benefit from home health care and more frequent intervention, including role-modeling to cope with disruptive and anxious behaviors.

Anxiety as a Protective Factor

Children and adolescents with conduct problems may show poor skills in identifying others' emotions and processing emotions of others, as measured through facial recognition tasks (Marsh & Blair, 2008). Interestingly, having a comorbid anxiety disorder may mitigate this effect. Short, Sonuga-Barke, Adams, and Fairchild (2016) assessed facial emotion recognition in groups of adolescents (12–18 years) with anxiety, CD, and CD + anxiety compared to controls. One requirement for participation in their study was having relatively higher levels of cognitive functioning (IQ equal to or above 75). Short et al. (2016) surmised that youth with CD would not recognize disgust, surprise, fear, sadness, and distress for others as well as youth who did not have conduct problems. They noted that children with anxiety might be more sensitive to "threat" types of emotions, like facial expressions of fear, sadness, and disgust. Youth completed a variety of facial recognition of emotion tasks, and results indicated that children with CD and anxiety performed more like controls, indicating that having comorbid anxiety provided a protective influence on emotion recognition. Hence, having anxiety was potentially an asset, as it was related to better recognition of "upset" emotionsin others. Irrespective of whether the children had an anxiety disorder, children with CD did tend to see neutral faces as sad, indicating that practice and skills in understanding others' emotions may be potential interventions for children with CD (Short et al., 2016).

Sonuga-Barke, Cortese, Fairchild, and Stringaris (2017) suggested that decision-making differs between children with conduct problems and anxiety. They described decision-making in children with conduct problems as tending to be reckless and insensitive to negative consequences. If this is the case, then perhaps the reduced novelty seeking associated with having anxiety (Melegari et al., 2015) helps youth hesitate and stay removed from some high-risk situations in which their insensitivity to the possibility of negative consequences could put them in harm's way. Sonuga-Barke et al. (2017) described children with anxiety as being hesitant, risk-aversive, and self-deprecating. If children with conduct problems and anxiety have a self-deprecating quality, maybe this quality is protective because others might not see behavior as "purposeful" if children were likely to take responsibility for it. On the other hand, Blair et al. (2014) reported that children with conduct problems and anxiety may not exhibit callous and unemotional traits, and anxiety serves as a protective factor against engaging in high-risk behavior that disregards the rights of others. These ideas are speculative and more research is needed to see if anxiety is a protective factor, at least for some populations with conduct problems and anxiety.

Anxiety as a Risk Factor

Conversely, Euler et al. (2015) reported anxiety may not be a protective factor for youth with conduct problems who have psychopathology and are likely to engage in high levels of violations against others. They may have higher levels of externalizing and other negative behaviors and be much less sensitive to the rights of others. Euler et al. (2015) examined callous and unemotional traits and negative behaviors in youth with CD and anxiety who were placed in the juvenile justice system or the foster care system. These youth were more likely to be in a subgroup exhibiting lower rates of prosocial behaviors—perhaps because they have experienced higher levels of trauma. Euler et al. (2015) measured several behaviors (e.g., externalizing problems) and traits/temperament for youth in their study. They used cluster analyses to group traits and behaviors for boys and girls. Their findings confirmed their hypotheses that there were higher levels of callous and unemotional traits in youth with higher levels of pathology and CD and anxiety symptoms. Moreover, they found that girls with CD, callous–unemotional traits, and anxiety reported higher levels of problematic, negative behaviors compared to boys. They proposed that their findings were preliminary, as their participants were in the welfare and/or juvenile justice systems. Hence, Euler et al. (2015) suggested that anxiety might not protect children and adolescents against callous traits, which is in contrast to ideas discussed by Blair et al. (2014). The jury is still out about whether anxiety is a protective or risk factor for youth.

Worrying on a daily basis can influence anxiety and possibly externalizing symptoms in youth. As such, repetitive worries or ruminating about worries regularly may be a risk factor for psychopathology in youth (Arbel, Perrone, & Margolin, 2018). Specifically, youth who engage in rumination about worries may seek relief or solace in substance use. In turn, they may engage in risky behaviors, if they are high in sensation seeking (and have conduct problems) as a means of escape from worry. Interestingly, anxiety may predict engaging in risky behavior for males but not females (Arbel et al., 2018). Nevertheless, support seeking can be a buffer, if the nature of social support is positive. Arbel et al. (2018) discovered that positive social support, from friends or family, could be a buffer against negative behaviors for youth with a pattern of risky behaviors and anxiety. Then again, if the nature of support was negative, and not perceived as supportive, then the opposite could occur, and youth could be a pushed toward acting in high-risk ways. The negative support could propel youth to engage in higher levels of worry, causing more risk behavior, and a potential negative cycle could occur. Arbel et al. (2018) did not differentiate between "who" provided the support, and thus they could not differentiate whether it was friends or family who were positive influences. Arbel et al. (2018) noted that clinicians need to ask adolescents about the nature of support they receive from others. If it is negative, finding positive sources of support for the youth may be a necessary component of therapy.

Chronic stress may influence the expression of externalizing problems and anxiety. Conway, Hammen, and Brennan (2012) found that chronic stress was linked to mental health problems, including internalizing and externalizing symptoms in youth. Snyder, Young, and Hankin (2019) reviewed the relationship between chronic stress and internalizing problems (among them anxiety) and externalizing problems in 567 youth in the third, sixth, and ninth grades (mean age about 15 years) in public schools in New Jersey and Denver. A screening criterion was cognitive functioning or an IQ score of over 70. Measurement intervals were at a baseline, 18 months and

36 months. Snyder et al. (2019) examined child functioning from baseline (Time 1) to 18 months (Time 2) to 36 months (Time 3). Participants completed measures to assess chronic stress and mental health problems, including a behavior problems checklist and anxiety scale. Snyder et al. (2019) reported that higher stress at Time 1 was related to higher levels of externalizing behaviors at Time 2. As expected, stress was independently correlated with anxiety. For older youth, academic stressors and stress related to experiencing violence were related to levels of mental health problems and psychopathology, indicating that screening for chronic stress in these areas is a goal for clinicians. Thus, Snyder et al. (2019) reported two pathways for chronic stress—it impacted general levels of pathology in youth and specifically acted on externalizing symptoms.

Anger for Children Who Experience Anxiety

Many children and adolescents with anxiety experience anger, irrespective of whether they have conduct problems. In a sample of youth with anxiety disorders, Johnco et al. (2015) reported that 55% of their sample experienced significant anger, which they called rage. A little over a third experienced rage symptoms at moderate levels of intensity. These researchers noted rage is common in anxiety disorders and does tend to dissipate over the course of treatment, as anxiety symptoms improve. Symptoms of rage have been associated with increased internalizing and externalizing problems (i.e., increased psychiatric symptomatology) and families accommodating the child's behaviors (Johnco et al., 2015). Parents and family should intervene when children who have anxiety become very angry so that they can learn appropriate emotion regulation skills. It is noteworthy that rage occurs for children with anxiety, and does not necessarily mean that the child has conduct problems. It may be that reactive aggression, related to frustration with behaviors and symptoms, underlies the expression of anger by some children with anxiety and conduct problems (Bubier & Drabick, 2009).

Emotion Dysregulation

The anger that children experience may be related to struggling with their anxiety disorder (Lebowitz, Storch, MacLeod, & Leckman, 2015). In turn, it may be related to emotion dysregulation. I define emotion regulation as coping appropriately with different emotions, especially upsetting ones. Schneider, Arch, and Landy (2018) reviewed the link between emotion dysregulation, which may be conceptualized as managing and changing emotions, and anxiety. They noted that repetitive worry may be a type of emotion dysregulation. Schneider et al. (2018) discussed emotional awareness as central to reducing emotional lability (rapidly changing, perhaps uncontrolled emotions). Acceptance, monitoring and managing emotions is critical for healthy development, especially positive social development. Schneider et al. (2018) assessed anxiety and emotion regulation in a sample of 312 adolescents (41% males), average of about 11 and a half years (*SD* = 2.3; range 8–16 years). These researchers used surveys to assess child anxiety, depression and symptoms of emotion dysregulation. Their findings indicated that poor awareness of emotions and a lack of acceptance of emotions were associated with social anxiety. Difficulties with goal-directed behavior were related to general anxiety. A lack of emotional awareness and a lack of goal-directed behavior predicted anxiety. They found anxiety scores decreased over time for youth. Schneider et al. (2018) recommended that when children recognize strong emotions, goal-directed behavior can be pursued to help them cope with their emotions.

In a similar manner, emotion dysregulation may be related to aggression in youth with conduct problems, such as ODD, CD, and ADHD (Lochman, Powell, Whidby, & Fitzgerald, 2012). Emotional responses involving significant anger may be related to processing social information differently, within a negative frame. This negative frame involves thinking others have negative or hostile intentions or that when events unfold aggression and violence will occur (e.g., "the event is threatening, provocative, frustrating"; Lochman et al., 2012, p. 29). This type of hostile attribution bias was discussed as biased processing of social information (e.g., Dodge's model, Crick & Dodge, 1994). Negative social appraisals may influence the emotional reactions of children with conduct problems. If they see others as hostile, children may feel both anxiety and worry, display aggression, and have difficulty regulating their emotions. It is necessary to change these types of attributions and reactions, as significant aggression in children is related to criminal behavior, academic difficulties, and a lack of employment (Troop-Gordon, Gordon, Vogel-Ciernia, Lee, & Visconti, 2018). Troop-Gordon et al. (2018) recommended using attentional retraining techniques to assist aggressive youth in attending to relevant cues when processing social information. As such, youth need to learn and practice how to react appropriately to provocation (in provocative situations) and in negative social situations. They also need to learn and practice friendship skills and social skills that will help them interact with others in a variety of social situations.

Interventions

Before presenting a review of interventions, it is noteworthy that some of the studies addressed disruptive behaviors and anxiety separately (i.e., with different sets of interventions). Combining interventions may be helpful for treatment of comorbid disruptive behaviors and anxiety. This may save time and then the clinician can address presenting problems quickly. First, the clinician could decide which symptoms need to be treated. For anxiety, teaching relaxation, positive imagery and positive self-talk, and exposure are valuable interventions. Teaching parents to ignore and not accommodate anxiety and use gradual exposure to a feared event or stimulus, with rewards for positive coping, are often beneficial techniques. For disruptive behaviors, teaching parents to stop or reduce coercive cycles (i.e., negative parent–child interactions and exchanges) can be helpful in changing the tone of the parent–child relationship. Teaching parents to reinforce positive behavior is essential. Using reward charts and then adding response costs to reward charts (loss of points or privileges) can be a key component of interventions for some children. Teaching problem-solving steps can be a central facet of treatment, not only for disruptive behaviors but also for anxiety. I think that the problem-solving component for disruptive behaviors will need to focus on having children take the perspective of others and learn how to think about and cope with their feelings. These are some preliminary ideas about intervention, and I am certain that clinicians will have other ideas as they review information in this section of the chapter.

As previously mentioned, Lebowitz et al. (2015) discussed that children with anxiety may experience anger related to their condition. Similarly, children with disruptive behaviors may experience significant anger, which can lead to aggression toward others (Blair et al., 2014; American Psychiatric Association (DSM-V), 2013; Kazdin, 1997). Lebowitz et al. (2015) recommended that when children recognize strong emotions, goal-directed behavior can be pursued to help them cope with their emotions. Being goal-directed to reduce anxiety is a strong component of Kendall's "FEAR" model, which involves recognizing feelings ("F"; feeling fear or fright), understanding one's expectations ("E"; Am I expecting bad things to happen?), attitudes and acting ("A" change negative thoughts and act positively to reduce negative feelings and avoidance of anxiety-provoking events and stimuli), and then rewarding oneself for coping with one's fears ("R"; Kendall, 2012). The acting positively aspect of the model can be stressed and suggestions made to help youth learn to pursue positive goals.

I believe that the FEAR model (Kendall, 2012) can be adapted for anger and emotion dysregulation in this manner—recognizing angry feelings ("F"), checking one's expectations ("E"; examples of checking expectations are—Do I think that the other person is doing this on purpose? Am I giving the other person the benefit of the doubt? Do I expect a negative result?), acting positively ("A," can I stop and think, can I relax and problem-solve and not react in anger?), and then the child can praise (or reward) himself or herself or receive tangible rewards for dialing down the drama and coping positively. For the "A" step, positive self-talk might be, I will take a friendly approach (I can understand how this person is feeling and act in a friendly, fair, and kind way). Thus, the "A" part of the model could be a place for incorporating strategies for appropriate actions, such as friendship skills and conflict resolution skills, when a child feels provoked. The "E" in the FEAR model focuses on expectations. I believe that children with disruptive behaviors or conduct problems often need to change their expectations, albeit that this is often in a different manner than children experiencing anxiety. For the "E" step, changing expectations may involve cognitive training to understand that—maybe the person did not do this with hostile intent. Consequently, within the "E" and "A" steps of the model, children can learn attentional retraining and new ways of acting that will assist them interpersonally and improve their self-regulation (Troop-Gordon et al., 2018).

This paragraph reviews some key ideas for treatment techniques. As stated, the clinician may want to teach the child to give others the benefit of the doubt. And, teach the child to calm down and stop and think, and use "feelings" words, before reacting in anger or in a hostile way. The "E" part of the model may be a place to incorporate training in "new" or positive expectations about others and how one reacts to others (Troop-Gordon et al., 2018). Additionally, a second step at the "E" level would be to ask the child to look at the clues for my expectations—maybe the other child is just trying to participate in the group and not take my place. Hence, I can be friendly and not be angry, because this child is just trying to be a part of the group.

Telephone-Based Interventions Telephone interventions have been effective. For example, McGrath et al. (2011) reviewed the impact of telephone-based interventions for children with disruptive behavior problems (ODD and ADHD) and anxiety disorders. Inclusion criteria, in terms of child age, were somewhat younger for children with ODD (3–7 years) than ADHD (8–12 years), and anxiety (6–12 years). They discussed how difficult it is for families to come to treatment, mentioning that only about 15–30% of families receive timely mental health services for their child. McGrath et al. (2011) discussed the benefits of their "Strongest Families Intervention" to treat disruptive behaviors or anxiety disorders in youth. Interventions were delivered by a telephone coach, using role-play and education. The program consisted of 11 or 12 sessions followed by two follow-up "booster" telephone sessions.

Sessions for ODD and ADHD focused on the following topics:

- Boosting good parent–child relationships by catching the child's good behavior,
- Ignoring negative behaviors (e.g., complaining),
- Use of transition warnings,
- Use of "when you do this, then that" type of statements,
- Teaching parents to have plans in place for negative behavior at home,
- Use of reward charts (with consequences [e.g., loss of points] for negative behaviors, and
- Working with staff at schools (McGrath et al., 2011).

Sessions for parents receiving education for children with *anxiety* included education about anxiety, such as: how it works in terms of triggers for fear, avoidance of the feared stimulus, and information about how the avoidance reinforces the anxiety making it stronger. Parents learned techniques that they could help their children use to reduce anxiety, such as the following:

- Muscle relaxation,
- Breathing,
- Imagery,
- Positive self-talk, and
- Gradual exposure to feared stimuli and events through role play (McGrath et al., 2011).

Finally, they discussed ideas for preventing relapse into the fear and avoidance cycles. Their findings indicated that children with disruptive behaviors or anxiety benefitted from telephone interventions, in terms of being diagnosis free, even after long-term follow-up (1 year; McGrath et al., 2011). However, each disorder was treated separately in their interventions. Unfortunately, they did not focus on comorbid presentations in treatment. Furthermore, their primary outcome was child diagnosis and measuring child functioning may have yielded more information about "how" the intervention was working. I believe that a modular approach for children with anxiety and ODD or ADHD, where lessons which focus on explanation of anxiety and interventions (muscle relaxation and breathing, imagery, exposure) are taught after the use of reward charts and application of interventions for disruptive behaviors, would benefit children with disruptive behaviors and anxiety. Clinicians could select interventions from the array of techniques to use to address presenting issues described earlier in this section. The effectiveness of these treatment techniques could be examined in an Internet-based program, which could reach a broad spectrum of clients.

Parent Involvement in Interventions Forehand, Jones, and Parent (2013) reviewed literature on parent involvement in interventions for anxiety or disruptive behaviors, with a focus on ODD and CD. They noted that parents can play a critical role in the treatment of disruptive behaviors. Moreover, if parents engage in patterns of coercive behaviors, then in a "cascading model" their behaviors can play a role in the development and enhancement of disruptive (aggressive and negative) behaviors in their child. This occurs when the child repeats the coercive behaviors with parents, teachers, and other children. They believed parent involvement in treating conduct problems can begin in preschool, and can focus on treatment of aggression and noncompliant behaviors (studies they reviewed showed children were between 2 and 9 years). Forehand et al. (2013) mentioned that parents were primary intervention agents in the treatment of disruptive behaviors. Parents should learn to use time-out procedures and ignoring, while praising positive behaviors among other techniques. Moreover, parents play a vital role in teaching their preschool-age child to communicate and problem-solve when a child is engaging in disruptive behaviors. Parents needed to increase positive role-modeling and provide rewards for positive, prosocial behaviors for children, while decreasing any coercive or negative behaviors children might be displaying.

Likewise, Forehand et al. (2013) suggested parents can play a role in treatment of anxiety, finding that involving parents improved interventions. Forehand et al. mentioned that parent involvement in treatment of anxiety usually occurs in later years (e.g., 7–14 years), beginning in elementary school. I would note that the exception to this might be separation anxiety and some instances of Generalized Anxiety Disorder, where parent involvement in treatment may occur at younger ages. When treating anxiety, Forehand et al. (2013) mentioned that parents might need to be less controlling of the child's behavior, while providing positive attention to appropriate behaviors. Parents should work on reinforcing nonanxious behavior and ignoring anxiety when possible. Since parent involvement can be critical to child success, developing modular interventions to improve parent involvement in the treatment of comorbid anxiety and disruptive behaviors may assist children in obtaining better outcomes. To this end, clinicians can continue to teach parents to praise appropriate behaviors and ignore those that are not appropriate. They can teach parents to use reinforcement appropriately and recognize they are "role models" of positive and prosocial behaviors for their children.

Chase and Eyberg (2008) tested an intervention for children with ODD and Separation Anxiety Disorder (SAD). They discussed literature showing SAD can actually increase externalizing behaviors in children. Their sample was drawn from a group of 64 children (3–6 years, mean age = 4.48, *SD* = 1.13) with ODD, and of this group—15 had comorbid SAD. The children with SAD did not differ from the other children on demographic variables, like child gender and age. The children were receiving Parent Child Interaction Therapy (PCIT). In this training, therapists typically work with parents, often side-by-side, to role model appropriate parenting behaviors. They can coach parents through a microphone or "a bug in the ear." They teach parents how to promote positive behaviors, use praise, and engage in nondirective play with the child, which can promote positive parent–child interactions. During nondirective (or child-directed) play parents used "... positive attending skills, such as reflecting the child's verbalizations and giving labeled praise" (Chase & Eyberg, 2008, p. 277). For example, a parent could act as a sport commentator, commenting on the child's "play product" saying, "I like how you stacked the blocks so tall." After learning the child-directed play skills, parents learned positive discipline skills—such as use of specific praise for following instructions and use of time-out for noncompliant behaviors. Interestingly, findings did not confirm that children with SAD displayed higher levels of behavior problems than children who did not have comorbid SAD. Results indicated that ODD symptoms decreased for children in both groups (i.e., those children with ODD and those with both ODD and SAD). Children with SAD had significant reductions in anxiety at post-treatment. In general, internalizing symptoms (as assessed on a behavior checklist) improved for both groups. Thus, the PCIT assisted in reducing symptoms, and moving the children toward improved behaviors and parent–child exchanges.

Mindfulness Snyder et al. (2019) found a link between stress, anxiety, and conduct problems. Children and adolescents whose parents are coercive may experience chronic, toxic stress. Perry-Parrish, Copeland-Linder, Webb, and Sibinga (2016) proposed that toxic stress can be related to emotion dysregulation in youth, and that overexposure to stress may lead to a breakdown in coping skills. Perry-Parrish et al. (2016) recommended mindfulness training, with a focus on the present and awareness of one's emotions and state of arousal in the present. This type of training may assist children or adolescents coping with toxic stress achieve better regulation of their emotions. They wrote that

> Mindfulness instruction is intended to enhance an individual's innate ability to be aware of what is happening internally and externally with open curiosity and without judgment (Perry-Parrish et al., 2016, p. 172).

Mindfulness interventions could be a component of treatments for comorbid conduct problems and anxiety, because children may be reactive and need to be present and evaluate their emotions from a distance. If they "stand back" from emotions, they can better engage in problem-solving. Mindfulness interventions could be focused on meditation, with children learning to focus on their breathing as they stop and relax. In terms of the "FEAR" model (Kendall, 2012), the practice of meditation or focus on breathing could come after the recognition of angry or highly anxious feelings.

Training parents on mindfulness and teaching them to coach, and then practice mindfulness with their child, can help parent and child to be present, triumph over emotion dysregulation, and be in a calmer state to access problem-solving strategies. Perry-Parrish et al. (2016) reviewed the literature for youth residing in urban areas where there can be high levels of violence and stress. They reported that mindfulness-based interventions resulted in reduced stress, behavior problems, feelings of self-hostility, and somatization. Similarly, children could exhibit improvements in optimism and self-regulation, with reduced depression and aggression. Teaching youth to meditate, with a focus on breathing and relaxation, could help them to "center" themselves emotionally, and be a critical component of modular interventions. Reviewing what is happening without judgment could help children deal with hostile or negative attributional biases that could be "setting" factors for aggressive and anxious behaviors (Lochman et al., 2012; Troop-Gordon et al., 2018). I believe that mindfulness training could be a fundamental component of modular treatment designs, and that this training could be a part of modules focusing on anxiety and disruptive behaviors.

Modular Interventions I have learned more about MATCH treatment from review of Chorpita and Weisz's (2009) book entitled, "*MATCH-ADTC: Modular Approach to Therapy for Children with Anxiety, Depression, Trauma, or Conduct Problems*." This approach features cognitive-behavioral interventions and parent training. With the MATCH protocol, a series of treatments follows after identifying a treatment target, by focusing on the initial presenting problems. The *MATCH-ADTC* book has flowcharts to guide treatment, worksheets, and guidelines for using evidence-based interventions (Chorpita & Weisz, 2009). The *MATCH-ADTC* book and programs usually rely on a dashboard and suggested measures so that clinicians may assess and track child progress over the course of treatment.

Weisz et al. (2012) noted that anxiety, conduct problems, and depression are priority conditions on a global scale. They tested both modular and standard treatment approaches in a well-controlled study. Youth in their sample (174 children and adolescents between 7 and 13 years, mean age of about 10 years) had sought outpatient treatment for anxiety, depression, or disruptive behavior problems. They used their modular "MATCH" Treatment (standardized, evidence-based treatment for each of the three disorders) compared to treatment as usual in the community. Clinicians in the MATCH condition used a collection of evidence-based procedures. These researchers used a behavioral checklist and child report of symptoms to measure progress, among other measures (Weisz et al., 2012). Findings demonstrated that children receiving modular treatment showed improved behaviors compared to those in a treatment as usual group.

Combining modules from *Defiant Children* (Barkley, 2013) and Coping Cat protocols (which uses the FEAR approach, Kendall, 2012) would be effective in treating anxiety and ODD/CD in children. Russell Barkley (2013) developed the, "*Defiant Children: A Clinician's Manual for Assessment and Parent Training* (*Third Edition*)"; this is a recent edition, but the interventions have been used for several years. This training centers on learning to be positive with the child, interacting positively with the child, using rewards and praise, and learning appropriate discipline techniques (including consequences, like response costs for negative behaviors). In many ways these interventions may be similar to those outlined by Chase and Eyberg (2008). I think that the clinician would treat the most prominent presenting problems first and then move between protocols for anxiety (Kendall, 2012) and disruptive behaviors (Barkley, 2013) based on the child's needs.

Chorpita et al. (2017) implemented modular treatment in California, as part of the "Child STEPs in California" program. They examined the modular approach (e.g., Chorpita & Weisz, 2009) versus other evidence-based treatments implemented in community mental health centers to treat depression, trauma, anxiety, and disruptive behaviors. Children in their study were between 5 and 15 years of age ($n = 138$ youth, 76 boys with a mean age of about 9 years; ethnically diverse sample). The study was administered in Los Angeles County in the United States, amidst a large-scale trial of use of evidence-based treatments for youth (the Department of Mental Health had required evidence-based treatments be used in mental health centers for reimbursement). Therapists assigned to the community group delivered their treatments as usual, using evidence-based interventions to meet the reimbursement requirement. Therapists in the MATCH group used MATCH interventions, focusing on evidence-based cognitive-behavioral techniques. Interventions included but were not limited to "… exposure, problem-solving, rewards, time out, cognitive restructuring (replacing negative with positive self-talk, for example), and relaxation" (Chorpita et al., 2017, p. 19). These researchers stressed fitting the treatment to the child's problems and utilizing parents as codesigners of interventions. Results indicated children showed improvement in symptoms and greater gains in positive functioning. Moreover, children in the MATCH group improved faster (demonstrating shorter treatment duration) than those in the community group. Although results were not statistically significant (probably due to the smaller number of children using medication), youth in the MATCH group showed less need for psychotropic medications than children in the community group.

Case Study

Jax is a 9-year-old boy with very disruptive and angry behaviors and anxiety. He is a competitive soccer and baseball player. He attends one of the best private schools in the city. Yet, he has trouble completing his work. He tends to become worried about his performance, at school, sports, and home, and then he explodes. He can be oppositional and defy his parents' requests. His angry behavior has disrupted the family. His two brothers are not receiving the attention they deserve. It was taking "all of his parents' time" to react to his negative behaviors. He threw food at his mother in the car and regularly threw objects at his brothers. He recently lost his temper at a soccer game. His father reported that other parents noted that "he does this all the time." After this, his mother and father became very worried about his behaviors. The same type of behavior was occurring for baseball, as Jax could become very upset if he "struck out."

Jax and his mother described his explosions as coming out of the blue and being "uncontrollable." Therapy began with building rapport through playing card games. Jax was wary of treatment, feeling that going to therapy was a signal he was not a "good" child and the cause of trouble within his family. As rapport was built, the therapist provided education about how anxiety and anger work in the body. The therapist discussed the need to reset one's system when upset feelings were occurring. Jax had previously participated in mindfulness training, focusing on breathing, with another therapist. After contacting Jax's previous therapist, this became a cornerstone of treatment. Jax really liked breathing and listening to soft music, which the therapist added as an intervention. Jax was able to relax and listen to music for 10 min per day. Twenty minutes was the recommended dose of relaxation, but Jax was not able to attain this goal.

Jax learned about the anxiety to anger link. For Jax, this link operated through control. He believed that if he had worked hard in sports or had been behaving fairly well at home, then things should go his way. The therapist explained, through using sports as an example, that one can put in hard work and be performing well, and perhaps a mistake can occur or everything does not go as planned. Jax and his therapist discussed his thinking as being erroneous, because a person cannot control everything that happens at a soccer or baseball game.

His therapist and Jax discussed how anger affected him. Jax gained insight into the fact that, when he got very angry, his athletic performance greatly deteriorated, and therefore he "lost" chances to show the progress he was making as an athlete. Jax identified that not having control of the outcome of sporting events really bothered him. The therapist and Jax processed that he could not necessarily have control of the outcome of sports or always be able to exhibit his "perfect" performance. They identified factors out of his control, such as the other boys' performances. They talked about how athletes do not, "perform their best every time," and sometimes athletes need to work through a day when their performance is not as strong as usual. They used Kendall's (2012) FEAR model to identify feelings (worry, rage), expectations (I have to perform perfectly), actions (breathe, reset, refocus on my sport and my joy related to my sport), and reward (praise myself or go for ice-cream after a good athletic performance). Jax worked to change his self-expectations to recapture the joy of kicking a soccer ball and swinging a bat. He was able to successfully identify feelings and expectations and began to act more positively at athletic events. He continued relaxation at home. He recognized being tired was a trigger for him to become upset easily. Thus, he learned he would need to use his relaxation and talk himself through situations, when he was feeling tired.

For Jax's parents, sessions focused on key tenets of PCIT (Chase & Eyberg, 2008) and *Defiant Children* (Barkley, 2013). His parents worked to reestablish a positive relationship with Jax, through use of praise for positive actions ("catching him being good") and a reward chart, where Jax received treats for having a "calm and kind day" at home. They reestablished their positive relationship with Jax through game play, walks, and bike rides in the neighborhood. They learned to encourage Jax to use positive self-talk, breathing, and muscle relaxation, if he became nervous at sports events.

After a period of 3 weeks, spent refocusing on positive interactions at home, his parents began to learn discipline techniques (e.g., how to use "time-out" and response costs). A time-out involved sitting on the steps at home for 9 min. During a time-out there was not any talking with others. After a timer rang, Jax had a chance to return to what he was doing and work things out or get them right. If this did not work, Jax went to his room to relax. Jax came back to have another try at positive behavior after time-out in his room. His parents learned about response cost—for verbal or physical aggression he would lose iPad privileges for 2 h. Jax came up with this response cost in an interactive session with his parents. Jax and his parents developed a reward chart, where Jax earned positive points for good behavior and for "holding in" or not displaying tantrums or verbal or physical aggression when he was angry. Likewise, response costs and time-outs were tallied and tracked on his reward chart. He had weekly meetings over ice cream to talk about improving his behavior with his parents. In a private session, his parents learned to use ignoring and learned anxiety management strategies. After a 7-week course of treatment, Jax had stopped using physical aggression at home. His use of verbally aggressive behaviors, such as name-calling, had reduced. There were no longer problems at sporting events. Jax reported decreased anxiety and the ability to, "control my temper, sometimes." Consequently, this treatment was fairly successful and utilized techniques for anxiety management and for decreasing disruptive behaviors to improve child functioning.

Conclusions

This chapter reviews ideas for conceptualizing conduct problems (chiefly ODD and CD) and anxiety in children and adolescents. It is not yet certain if anxiety is protective in the expression of disruptive and antisocial behaviors for children who have conduct problems, and more research in this area is needed. Children who experience anxiety can express rage and anger, so differential diagnosis, to determine if behaviors reach the level of concern for conduct problems will guide the selection of treatment targets. Understanding feelings, changing expectations, and positive actions may be tools for addressing emotion dysregulation due to worry or anger. Teaching problem-solving using the FEAR model (Kendall, 2012) may be an intervention technique that can treat both disruptive and anxious symptoms. If conduct problems are severe, they may need to be addressed prior to treatment of anxiety. Involving parents in treatment, and stressing improving parent–child interactions to reduce coercive cycles, may change interaction patters and allow the child to model positive behaviors displayed by parents. Beginning with positives (reward charts and positive interactions), and then moving to consequences, such as time-out and response cost, is recommended. Telephone- and Internet-based interventions to reach large groups may be a wave of the future, allowing clinicians to educate more clients and parents.

References

American Psychiatric Association (DSM-V). (2013). *Diagnostic and statistical manual of mental disorders* (5th ed.). Washington, DC: Author.

Arbel, R., Perrone, L., & Margolin, G. (2018). Adolescents' daily worries and risky behaviors: The buffering role of support seeking. *Journal of Clinical Child and Adolescent Psychology, 47*(6), 900–911. https://doi.org/10.1080/15374416.2016.1169536

Barkley, R. A. (2013). *Defiant children: A clinician's manual for assessment and parent training* (3rd ed.). New York: Guilford.

Blair, R. J. R., Leibenluft, E., & Pine, D. S. (2014). Conduct disorder and callous–Unemotional traits in youth. *New England Journal of Medicine, 371*(23), 2207–2216. https://doi.org/10.1056/NEJMra1315612

Bubier, J. L., & Drabick, D. A. G. (2009). Co-occurring anxiety and disruptive behavior disorders: The roles of anxious symptoms, reactive aggression, and shared risk processes. *Clinical Psychology Review, 29*(7), 658–669. https://doi.org/10.1016/j.cpr.2009.08.005

Chase, R. M., & Eyberg, S. M. (2008). Clinical presentation and treatment outcome for children with comorbid externalizing and internalizing symptoms. *Anxiety Disorders, 22*, 273–282. https://doi.org/10.1016/j.anxdis2007.03.006

Chorpita, B. F., Daleiden, E. L., Park, A. L., Ward, A. M., Levy, M. C., Cromley, T., … Krull, J. L. (2017). Child STEPs in California: A cluster randomized effectiveness trial comparing modular treatment with community implemented treatment for youth with anxiety, depression, conduct problems, or traumatic stress. *Journal of Consulting and Clinical Psychology, 85*(1), 13–25. https://doi.org/10.1037/ccp0000133

Chorpita, B. F., & Weisz, J. R. (2009). *MATCH-ADTC: Modular approach to therapy for children with anxiety, depression, trauma, or conduct problems*. Satellite Beach, FL: PracticeWise, LLC.

Conway, C. C., Hammen, C., & Brennan, P. A. (2012). Expanding stress generation theory: Test of a transdiagnostic model. *Journal of Abnormal Psychology, 121*, 754–766. https://doi.org/10.1037/a0027457

Crick, N. R., & Dodge, K. A. (1994). A review and reformulation of social information-processing mechanisms in children's social adjustment. *Psychological Bulletin, 115*, 74–101. https://doi.org/10.1037/0033-2909.115.1.74

Euler, F., Jenkel, N., Stadler, C., Schmeck, K., Fegert, J. M., … Schmid, M. (2015). Variants of girls and boys with conduct disorder: Anxiety symptoms and callous-unemotional traits. *Journal of Abnormal Child Psychology, 43*(4), 773–785. https://doi.org/10.1007/s10802-014-9946-x

Forehand, R., Jones, D. J., & Parent, J. (2013). Behavioral parenting interventions for child disruptive behaviors and anxiety: What's different and what's the same. *Clinical Psychology Review, 33*(1), 133–145. https://doi.org/10.1016/j/cpr.2012.10.010

Johnco, C., Salloum, A., De Nadai, A. S., McBride, N., Crawford, E. A., Lewin, A. B., & Storch, E. A. (2015). Incidence, clinical correlates and treatment effect of rage in anxious children. *Psychiatry Research, 229*, 63–69. https://doi.org/10.1016/j.psychres.2015.07.071

Kazdin, A. E. (1997, February). Practitioner review: Psychosocial treatments for conduct disorder in children. *Journal of Clinical Psychology and Psychiatry, 38*(2), 161–178. https://doi.org/10.1111/j.1469-7610.1997.tb01851.x. downloaded on August 4, 2019.

Kendall, P. C. (2012). Anxiety disorders in youth. In P. C. Kendall (Ed.), *Child and adolescent therapy: Cognitive-behavioral procedures* (4th ed., pp. 143–189). New York, NY: Guilford.

Lebowitz, E. R., Storch, E. A., MacLeod, J., & Leckman, J. F. (2015). Clinical and family correlates of coercive-disruptive behavior in children and adolescents with obsessive-compulsive disorder. *Journal of Child and Family Studies, 24*(9), 2589–2597. https://doi.org/10.1007/s10826-014-0061-y

Lochman, J. E., Powell, N. P., Whidby, J. M., & FitzGerald, D. P. (2012). Aggression in children. In P. C. Kendall (Ed.), *Child and adolescent therapy: Cognitive-behavioral procedures* (4th ed., pp. 27–60). New York, NY: Guilford.

Marsh, A. A., & Blair, R. J. R. (2008). Deficits in facial affect recognition among antisocial populations: A meta-analysis. *Neuroscience and Behavioral Reviews, 32*(3), 454–465. https://doi.org/10.1016/j.neubiorev.2007.08.003

McGrath, P. J., Lingley-Pottie, P., Thurston, C., MacLean, C., Cunningham, C., Waschbusch, D. A., … Chaplin, W. (2011). Telephone-based mental health interventions for child disruptive behavior or anxiety disorders: Randomized trials and overall analysis. *Journal of the American Academy of Child and Adolescent Psychiatry, 50*(11), 1162–1172. https://doi.org/10.1016/j.jaac.2011.07.013

Melegari, M. G., Nani, V., Lucidi, F., Russo, P. M., Donfrancesco, R., & Cloninger, R. (2015). Temperamental and character profiles of preschool children with ODD, ADHD, and anxiety disorders. *Comprehensive Psychiatry, 58*, 94–101. https://doi.org/10.1016/j.comppsych.2015.01.001

Perry-Parrish, C., Copeland-Linder, N., Webb, L., & Sibinga, E. (2016). Mindfulness-based approaches for children and youth. *Current Problems in Pediatric and Adolescent Health Care, 46*, 172–178. https://doi.org/10.1016/j.cppeds.2015.12.006

Schneider, R. L., Arch, J. J., & Landy, L. N. (2018). The longitudinal effect of emotion regulation strategies on anxiety levels in children and adolescents. *Journal of Clinical Child & Adolescent Psychology, 47*(6), 978–991. https://doi.org/10.1080/15374416.2016.1157757

Short, R. M. L., Sonuga-Barke, E. J. S., Adams, W. J., & Fairchild, G. (2016). Does comorbid anxiety counteract emotion regulation deficits in conduct disorder? *Journal of Child Psychology and Psychiatry, 57*(8), 917–926. https://doi.org/10.1111/jccp.12544

Snyder, H. R., Young, J. F., & Hankin, B. L. (2019). Chronic stress exposure and generation are related to the p-factor and externalizing specific to psychopathology in youth. *Journal of Clinical Child and Adolescent Psychology, 48*(2), 306–315. https://doi.org/10.1080/15374416.2017.1321002

Sonuga-Barke, E. J. S., Cortese, S., Fairchild, G., & Stringaris, A. (2017). Annual research review: Transdiagnostic neuroscience of child and adolescent mental disorders—differentiating decision making in attention-deficit/hyperactivity disorder, conduct disorder, depression, and anxiety. *Journal of Child Psychology and Psychiatry, 57*(3), 321–349. https://doi.org/10.1111/jcpp.12496

Storch, E. A., Arnold, E. B., Jones, A. M., Ale, C. M., Wood, J. J., Ehrenreich-May, J., … Murphy, T. K. (2012). The role of co-occurring disruptive behavior in the clinical presentation of children and adolescents with anxiety in the context of autism spectrum disorders. *Child Psychiatry & Human Development, 43*(5), 734–746. https://doi.org/10.1007/s10578-012-0294-1

Tolan, P. H., Dodge, K., & Rutter, M. (2013). Tracking the multiple pathways of parent and family influence on disruptive behavior disorders. In P. H. Tolan & B. L. Leventhal (Eds.), *Disruptive behavior disorders, advances in developmental psychopathology: Brain research foundation symposium series* (pp. 161–192). New York: Science+Business Media, Springer. https://doi.org/10.1007/978-1-4614-7557-6_7

Troop-Gordon, W., Gordon, R. D., Vogel-Ciernia, L., Lee, E. E., & Visconti, K. J. (2018). Visual attention to dynamic scenes of ambiguous provocation and children's aggressive behavior. *Journal of Clinical Child & Adolescent Psychology, 47*(6), 925–940. https://doi.org/10.1080/15374416.2016.1138412

Weisz, J. R., Chorpita, B. F., Palinkas, L. A., Schoenwald, S. K., Miranda, J., Bearman, S. K., … the Research Network on Youth Mental Health. (2012). Testing for standard and modular designs for psychotherapy treating depression, anxiety, and conduct problems in youth: A randomized effectiveness trial. *Archives of General Psychiatry, 69*(3), 274–282. https://doi.org/10.1001/archgenpsychiatry.2011.147

Chapter 9
Summary

Critical Ideas in This Book

As mentioned in the preface to this book, evidence-based treatments are using "what works" to assist children in their recovery. However, evidence-based treatments can take quite some time and resources to implement. Concomitantly, one's clients might not always have eight to ten sessions to work with a clinician, such as parents who are bringing their child for help using Employee Assistance Programs, where only three visits have been approved. Clinicians may need to make a difference quickly, and use of pieces of interventions, such as those suggested in modular approaches.

As such, a modular approach may be beneficial when clinicians are working with one child and his or her family (Chorpita & Weisz, 2009). Many clinicians practice using this model. Furthermore, it may be difficult to recruit children for group treatment, as many children and parents have busy schedules and cannot commit to a consistent weekly meeting time. It may be that clinicians working in private practice or community mental health settings do not have a significant number of children with similar symptoms on caseloads at the same time, making it difficult to introduce a group treatment. In these cases, individual treatment is needed. Clinicians take careful stock of presenting problems and work to address them. Parent and child reports, either through clinician interviews or responses on surveys, are typically used to measure child progress. The case studies and review of information in this book were meant to assist clinicians in thinking about working with children, adolescents, and parents using evidence-based cognitive-behavioral therapy (CBT) techniques to design individualized treatment plans to implement interventions to address children's and parents' chief concerns or most pressing presenting problems. The modular approach is consistent with a clinical approach, and assessing progress in terms of measuring symptom relief meets a primary purpose of therapy,

L. Nabors, *Anxiety Management in Children with Mental and Physical Health Problems*, Springer Series on Child and Family Studies,
https://doi.org/10.1007/978-3-030-35606-4_9

which is to improve or ease suffering (personal communication, Dr. Nirbhay Singh, May 6, 2019).

In many cases, the clinician will not be able to determine which disorder predates the child's problems. Similarly, although there is a genetic predisposition to many child and adolescent mental health problems, as of yet knowledge of genetics does not lead to a cure or remission of symptoms. Because the aforementioned information is indeterminate, it may not be needed to guide treatment. Needing to alleviate feelings of anxiety or behaviors that are not positive for the child are of immediate concern and addressing "concerning symptoms," which cause suffering, is a way to improve functioning for the child and indirectly improve family functioning as well. Helping alleviate the negative impact of problematic symptoms may engage parents, which can be essential as they are point persons for implementing treatment at home. Parents may also convey treatment ideas to teachers, when clinicians are not able to connect with them. Having an informed and involved parent can ensure that reward charts are used and time is taken to change family interaction patterns, contributing to the success of interventions. What is more, parents may experience anxiety, and helping them learn strategies to manage their symptoms and become positive role models for their child may further enhance treatment effects.

CBT techniques are relatively easy for parents, children, and adolescents to learn. Tracking observable behaviors, using charts on refrigerators and simple notebooks, is way that parents, children, and adolescents can check progress and decide if interventions are working or if they need to try another technique. Problem-solving and being a detective to find out what works and when it works is at the heart of making interventions work. Explaining to clients and parents that anxiety can "morph" and become different worries can help arm them against a relapse, or a return to "anxiety-driven responding." Explaining "Grandma's Cure," which is to move through anxiety-provoking situations and face one's fears and power through them, is at the heart of many treatments, including graded exposures to fearful situations or events. Using relaxation, positive self-statements, and positive imagery are other key interventions I have used with children and adolescents facing anxiety. These strategies, from a detective stance or problem-solving framework, can be modified to treat other problems, including anger (conduct problems) and upset (perhaps related to changing routines for children with Autism Spectrum Disorder). I have used Kendall's (2012) FEAR model, helping children identify feelings, change expectations, introduce positive actions, and reinforce their efforts to treat anxiety, behavior problems (e.g., anger), and a host of other problems. These techniques and other CBT interventions, when implemented within a positive psychology framework, appear to be one positive stance for approaching problems (Seligman & Csikszentmihalyi, 2000). Moving toward positive functioning alleviates suffering and, hopefully, can begin a positive developmental trajectory for clients.

Further research is needed to learn what works for whom. Learning what works for children in different age ranges, with different comorbid problems, is a way to expand knowledge about successful treatments. It may be that clinicians can "add knowledge" to the modular approach by writing about what works for children of different ages, with different types of presenting problems. Another idea for adding to our literature base is to encourage researchers and editors to publish more case studies so that we can gain more knowledge about how treatments are tailored to youth of different ages, with differing levels of symptom severity. Another area where more research is needed is applying interventions for youth with lower levels of cognitive functioning. Finding ways to apply CBT and ensure that training generalizes and whether interventions can "last" without reinforcement are areas for discovery related to working with children and adolescents with lower levels of cognitive functioning. Finally, do CBT techniques "fit" for families of all cultures? How can we implement techniques within a positive framework that is culturally appropriate? In reviewing literature to write this book, these are some of the questions that emerged. It is truly amazing to see how far the field has come in addressing mental health problems for children and adolescents. It was such a pleasure to review all the positive interventions and the wonderful treatments that could be implemented in schools. As clinicians move forward and move the field forward, it will be important to learn about how we can help more children and families, and tailor treatment to meet their needs to further improve emotional and behavioral functioning for children and adolescents.

References

Chorpita, B. F., & Weisz, J. R. (2009). *MATCH-ADTC: modular approach to therapy for children with anxiety, depression, trauma, or conduct problems*. Satellite Beach, FL: PracticeWise, LLC.

Kendall, P. C. (2012). Anxiety disorders in youth. In P. C. Kendall (Ed.), *Child and adolescent therapy: Cognitive-behavioral procedures* (4th ed., pp. 143–189). New York, NY: Guilford.

Seligman, M. E. P., & Csikszentmihalyi, M. (2000). Positive psychology: An introduction. *American Psychologist, 55*(1), 5–14. https://doi.org/10.1037/0003-066X.55.1.5 downloaded on August 4, 2019.

Index

L. Nabors, *Anxiety Management in Children with Mental and Physical Health Problems*, Springer Series on Child and Family Studies,
https://doi.org/10.1007/978-3-030-35606-4

The manufacturer's authorised representative in the EU is Springer Nature Customer Service Centre GmbH, Europaplatz 3, 69115 Heidelberg, Germany. If you have any concerns regarding our products, please contact ProductSafety@springernature.com

Printed and bound by CPI Group (UK) Ltd, Croydon, CR0 4YY

30/09/2026

02225574-0011